Pathology of Female Cancers

Takuya Moriya
Editor

Pathology of Female Cancers

Precursor and Early-Stage Breast, Ovarian and Uterine Carcinomas

Springer

Editor
Takuya Moriya
Department of Pathology
Kawasaki Medical School
Kurashiki
Japan

ISBN 978-981-10-8605-2　　ISBN 978-981-10-8606-9 (eBook)
https://doi.org/10.1007/978-981-10-8606-9

Library of Congress Control Number: 2018949328

Printed on acid-free paper

This Springer imprint is published by the registered company Springer Nature Singapore Pte Ltd.
The registered company address is: 152 Beach Road, #21-01/04 Gateway East, Singapore 189721, Singapore

Preface

Often, cancers are characterized by their abrupt occurrence. However, most cancers originate earlier and gradually develop in the subclinical stage. Even though this development varies from organ to organ, it may also differ for each patient. Hence, individualizing patients in terms of effective therapy and the early detection of cancer is imperative. Furthermore, the prevention of cancer is essential to avoid its proliferation.

Surgical pathologists are expected to provide a definitive diagnosis of cancer and precisely assess the biological behavior of each patient. However, the accurate diagnosis of precancerous lesions and the precise assessment of the possibility and their progression rate into clinically significant cancer will be spectacular, rendering the precancerous stage as entirely curable.

Apparently, the pathological diagnosis of all precancerous stages is complicated, as not all stages are morphologically evident. However, we may be able to detect precancerous "lesions." On the basis of the organs and/or histological types, the concept and term of these lesions vary, including dysplasia (i.e., uterine cervix), atypical hyperplasia (i.e., endometrium), adenoma (i.e., colorectum), intraepithelial neoplasia, or intraepithelial lesion. Occasionally, intraductal (noninvasive) carcinomas may also be included, as these are non-lethal and their distinction from dysplasia is complicated.

The primary feature of precancerous lesions is their potential to progress into definite (invasive) cancer in future, even though the possibility and their progression rates vary, leading to the use of the terms "borderline lesions," "borderline malignancy," or "atypically proliferating lesions" in some organs (e.g., ovary). Although benign and malignant tumors may possess a middle degree of atypia, their biological behavior (early stage and the possibility of progression) may not be necessarily considered. At times, the same technical term may be used differently; for example, atypical hyperplasia in the breast signifies risk lesions rather than real precursors, and adenomas in various organs are entirely benign that will not progress into adenocarcinoma. Furthermore, several cancers may not have precursors and directly originate from healthy tissues (de novo cancer).

This textbook intends to elucidate the current standards and novel knowledge regarding carcinogenesis, molecular features, histopathological diagnosis, and the clinical significance of precancerous and early-stage female cancers such as breast, ovarian, and uterine carcinomas. Apparently, the pathways of cancer development significantly vary among organs, with heterogeneous precursors and early lesions based on the histological type of cancer in the same organ. Recently, several paradigm shifts have been advocated in these areas, for examples, the underlying mechanism of high-grade serous carcinoma of the ovary (and the peritoneum). It may be reckoned that the recognition of the current concept will lead to the most appropriate approach for the diagnosis, treatment, and patient care.

As readers of this book may be familiar with the variegated development of these cancers, this book comprises eight chapters, including two chapters focusing on uterine cervical (precursors of squamous cell carcinoma and adenocarcinoma), one on endometrial (heterogeneity of precursors), three on ovarian (two pathways of carcinogenesis and the significance of borderline tumors), and two on mammary (significance of intrinsic subtype and risk assessment for non-cancerous lesions) cancers.

All contributors to this book are exceptional Japanese surgical pathologists. Although each chapter in this book puts forth global perspectives, it also presents Japanese perspective in some parts. I hope that this book serves as a useful reference for grasping the advanced knowledge and facilitate the daily practice of pathologists, gynecologists, breast surgeons, and all medical staff members in these fields.

Kurashiki, Japan Takuya Moriya

Contents

1 A New Strategy for Diagnosing of Squamous Intraepithelial Neoplasia of the Cervix

Yoshiki Mikami

Abstract

In 2014 the World Health Organization classification of female genital tract tumors was revised and published to employ the histopathologic term squamous intraepithelial lesion (SIL), which the Bethesda system had introduced to standardize cytology reporting in 1988. This revision reflects a paradigm shift in the views regarding the morphological and biological aspects of precancerous squamous lesions of the uterine cervix. Low-grade SIL is defined as productive human papillomavirus (HPV) infection, whereas high-grade SIL represents a neoplastic condition resulting from transformation owing to the integration of HPV DNA into the host genome. Currently, a variety of ancillary methods, including immunohistochemistry (IHC), contribute to establishing a correct diagnosis or optimal management for women with SIL. For example, a combination of Ki-67 and p16^{INK4a} IHC, as well as HPV IHC or in situ hybridization, is routinely used to facilitate diagnosis. In this chapter, current concepts, controversies, and diagnostic strategies for SIL are discussed.

Keywords

Uterine cervix · SIL · Precursor · Biomarker

1.1 Historical and Conceptual Aspects of Precancerous Squamous Lesions

Descriptions of the incipient phase of squamous cell carcinoma (SCC) of the uterine cervix appeared in the literature in the early twentieth century [1], and "carcinoma in situ," described by Broders in 1932 [2], has been recognized as a precancerous lesion. Thereafter, Reagan et al. coined the term "dysplasia" for intraepithelial lesions with a spectrum of cytologic abnormalities, ranging from mild to severe dysplasia, and to be distinguished from carcinoma in situ [3]. The term cervical intraepithelial neoplasia (CIN), currently used worldwide, was proposed by Richart in 1967 [4]. In this scheme, mild dysplasia and moderate dysplasia correspond to CIN 1 and CIN 2, respectively, and severe dysplasia and carcinoma in situ are lumped together as CIN 3. The rationale of this nomenclature is (1) suboptimal interobserver agreement regarding the distinction between severe dysplasia and carcinoma in situ, (2) frequent coexistence of these two conditions, and (3) similar risk of developing invasive carcinoma. Based on clinicopathological observations, CIN 1 is thought to progress to invasive carcinoma via CIN 2 and CIN 3 in a step-by-step fashion and in a timeframe ranging from 8 to 15 years. In 1983 human papillomavirus (HPV) was identified as a causative agent for developing cervical SCC [5].There is an implication for HPV infection in CIN, as well as for patients with condyloma, and the presence of koilocytosis, a morphologic expression of viral cytopathic effects, indicating that condyloma and CIN are included in the spectrum of HPV-driven squamous carcinogenesis [6–8].

In 1988, the Bethesda system (TBS) was introduced for standardization and quality management of cervical or vaginal smear cytology in the United States [9]. TBS proposed the term squamous intraepithelial lesion (SIL) and divided it into low-grade (LSIL) and high-grade (HSIL) categories. LSIL includes condyloma acuminatum and CIN 1, while HSIL includes CIN 2 and CIN 3, emphasizing that the distinction between CIN 1 and CIN 2/CIN 3 is crucial for patient management, because (1) the aim of TBS is to detect CIN 2 or more severe lesions, (2) condyloma and CIN 1 mostly regress or remain, and (3) interobserver agreement appeared optimal by drawing a line between CIN 1 and CIN 2.

Y. Mikami
Department of Diagnostic Pathology, Kumamoto Univerisity Hospital, Kumamoto, Kumamoto, Japan
e-mail: mika@kuhp.kyoto-u.ac.jp

T. Moriya (ed.), *Pathology of Female Cancers*, https://doi.org/10.1007/978-981-10-8606-9_1

Table 1.1 Classification of cervical squamous cell carcinoma precursors

<table>
<tr><th></th><th>Mild dysplasia</th><th>Moderate dysplasia</th><th>Severe dysplasia</th><th>Carcinoma in situ</th><th>Dysplasia-carcinoma in situ classification</th></tr>
<tr><td></td><td>CIN 1</td><td>CIN 2</td><td colspan="2">CIN 3</td><td>CIN classification</td></tr>
<tr><td>Condyloma</td><td>CIN 1</td><td>CIN 2</td><td colspan="2">CIN 3</td><td>Condyloma-CIN classification</td></tr>
<tr><td colspan="2">CIN 1</td><td>CIN 2</td><td colspan="2">CIN 3</td><td>WHO classification (1997)</td></tr>
<tr><td colspan="2">LSIL (cytology)</td><td colspan="3">HISL (cytology)</td><td>Bethesda system (1988)</td></tr>
<tr><td colspan="2">LSIL (histology)</td><td colspan="3">HSIL (histology)</td><td>WHO classification (2014)</td></tr>
</table>

In the following decade, SIL terminology became accepted for histopathologic diagnosis, and in 2012 the Lower Anogenital Squamous Terminology (LAST) consensus guideline, proposed by a collaboration of the College of American Pathologists (CAP) and the American Society of Colposcopy and Cervical Pathology (ASCCP), recommended SIL as a histopathologic term [10]. Consequently, the revised World Health Organization (WHO) classification (2014) supported the consensus [11].

The two-tiered system, i.e., LSIL/HSIL terminology, appears reasonable because (1) interobserver agreement among pathologists in distinguishing CIN 2 and CIN 3 is suboptimal [12, 13] and (2) both conditions share aneuploidy and genetic abnormalities, with a significant risk for developing invasive carcinoma. In other words, CIN 2 is not merely a biologically intermediate between CIN 1 and CIN 3; rather, it is closely related to CIN 3 or SCC. Therefore, a biopsy diagnosis of CIN 2 does not exclude the coexistence of CIN 3 and, thus, may not justify surveillance for the patient. In fact, the ASCCP guideline regards CIN 2 as a threshold for ablation therapy for women with HSIL diagnoses in the United States, although young and pregnant women can be monitored to avoid the risk of premature delivery related to conization [14]. Active surveillance for CIN 2 is considered acceptable in settings where accessibility to gynecologists specializing in colposcopy and the management for SIL patients is available. In this regard, the distinction between CIN 2 and CIN 3 may be crucial, and thus, the LAST guideline recommends using both systems. For example, the diagnostic note may be "HSIL/CIN 2" [10].

The WHO classification (2014) defines LSIL as the clinical and morphological manifestation of a productive HPV infection involving squamous epithelium, without significant risk for the coexistence or development of cancer. It should be kept in mind that even when the cytologic atypia is confined to the lower third of the epithelium, the lesion is designated as HSIL in case of significant cytologic atypia exceeding that of prototypical condyloma acuminatum, emphasizing the importance of abnormal mitotic figures, including tripolar or tetrapolar mitoses [11]. This is a departure from the traditional "one third" criteria, and a subset of intraepithelial lesions, which had been regarded as CIN 1, may now be reclassified as HSIL. A summary of these classification systems is shown in Table 1.1.

1.1.1 LSIL

As mentioned previously, LSIL is a productive HPV infection, showing cytopathic effects due to the replication of viral particles in the nuclei of superficial cells [15]. It is mostly a flat lesion and, thus, is also called "flat condyloma." "Mild squamous dysplasia," "CIN 1," "koilocytosis," and "koilocytotic atypia" are synonyms in the WHO classification (2014). The risk of progression to invasive carcinoma is low, and approximately 60% of LSIL regress, 30% persist, and 10% progress to HSIL due to the persistence of the infection. In approximately 80% of cases, high-risk HPV DNA, mostly types 16 or 18, is detected.

There are some controversies and confusions regarding the term LSIL. First, "flat condyloma" is considered to be an inappropriate term, since it conveys an erroneous impression that it is a condition biologically similar to condyloma acuminatum. Although both lesions are included in the LSIL category, "flat condyloma" is mostly a high-risk HPV-driven lesion, while condyloma acuminatum is associated with low-risk HPV, particularly types 6 and 11, has negligible risk for developing SCC, and, thus, is independently included in the benign squamous lesions in the WHO classification (2014). Therefore, the use of the term "flat condyloma" should be avoided. Second, "koilocytosis" or "koilocytotic atypia" is a microscopic finding rather than a disease entity that represents viral replication and is also identified in up to 50% of HSIL cases. This highlights the fact that these terms are not strictly synonyms of LSIL. Third, the WHO classification (2014) describes CIN 1 and LSIL as synonyms [15], but scientifically this view is incorrect because LSIL is by definition an infection, whereas semantically CIN 1 is a neoplastic condition. Actually, some pathologists may believe CIN 1 and HPV infection should be distinguished from each other for diagnostic purposes, but the LAST guideline and the WHO classification (2014) do not support this opinion, because (1) the distinctions based on morphology are challenging and not reproducible, (2) reliable discriminating biomarkers are absent, and (3) both conditions usually regress, and risk of progression is negligible [15, 16]. For clinical management purposes, it is much more important to distinguish LSIL from HSIL than subdividing LSIL.

LSIL is typically seen among women in their early 20s and with no significant clinical manifestations. The diagnosis is established by microscopic examination of biopsy specimens taken after cytologic interpretation of LSIL or atypical squamous cells of undetermined significance (ASC-US). In general, women with an LSIL diagnosis are monitored, but the interval of surveillance may be modified by HPV genotyping, as risk and interval for progression are influenced by HPV types.

Microscopically, LSIL is characterized by koilocytosis involving the superficial portion of the stratified squamous epithelium, which commonly shows hyperkeratosis or parakeratosis (Figs. 1.1 and 1.2). Individual keratinization and nuclear enlargement can be seen, but mitotic figures are scant and abnormal mitosis is uncommon. Koilocytosis should be strictly defined as features representing cytopathic effects due to viral replication in the nuclei of prickle cells, i.e., nuclear enlargement, heterogeneity in nuclear size and shape, nuclear irregularity ("raisinoid" nuclear contour), ground-glass or smudgy nuclear appearance, and perinuclear halos. The halo is well demarcated, and the periphery of the cytoplasm appears dense. Nuclear size may be 3–4 times larger than neighboring cells. Furthermore, multi- or binucleation is common, although a recent three-dimensional reconstruction study demonstrated that it represents hyper-lobulation [17].

The differential diagnosis includes reactive squamous atypia and HSIL. The former is distinguished from LSIL by the absence of koilocytosis, but frequently it is difficult to assess, because in the involutional phase of HPV infection, classic features of koilocytosis disappear from the surface of the epithelium. Pseudokoilocytosis or cytoplasmic clearing due to an accumulation of glycogen might be a source of misinterpretation. As explained below, HPV immunohistochemistry (IHC) or in situ hybridization (ISH) may contribute to establishing an LSIL diagnosis. $p16^{INK4a}$ IHC may contribute in some positive cases, but for the majority of cases, it is of limited value because only 30% of LSILs are positive for this marker. HSIL is distinguished from LSIL by significant nuclear abnormalities exceeding those of condyloma acuminatum. Nuclear hyperchromasia, heterogeneity in nuclear size and shape, and overlapping nuclei, as well as abnormal mitoses including tripolar mitosis, justify an HSIL diagnoses, even when these features are confined to the lower third of the epithelium (Fig. 1.3).

A minor subset of LSIL may coexist with HSIL, and such a condition may represent (1) LSIL progressing to HSIL or (2) the collision of two lesions caused by different types of

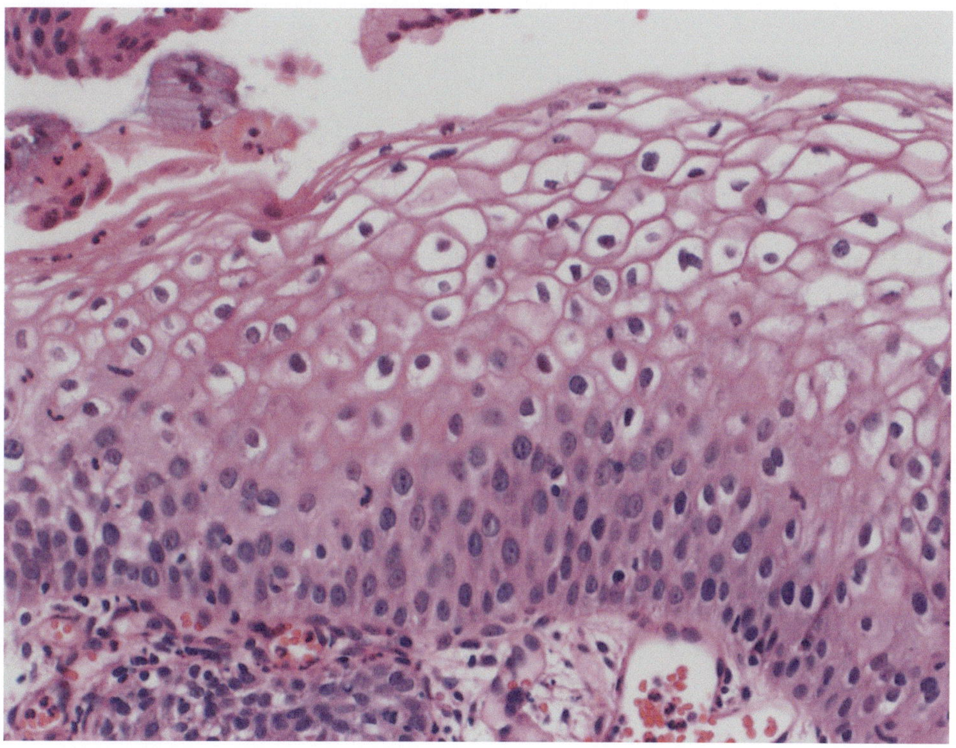

Fig. 1.1 LSIL (CIN 1) showing minimal cytologic atypia in the basal side and koilocytosis in the upper side

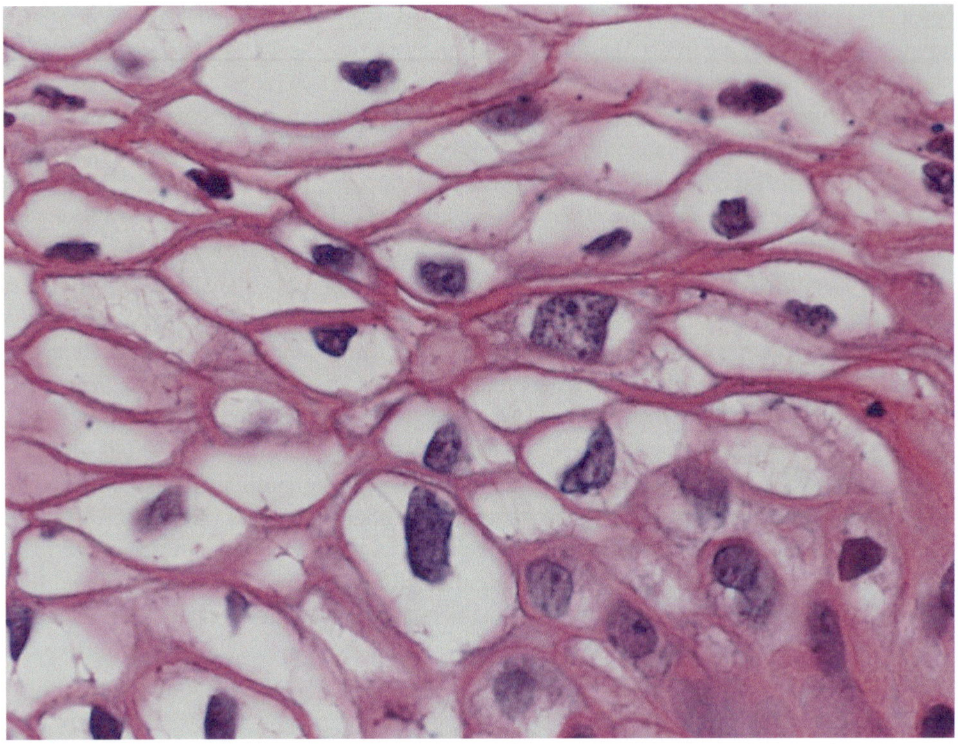

Fig. 1.2 LSIL (CIN 1) with koilocytosis, characterized by irregularity in nuclear shapes and sizes, showing a perinuclear halo with a sharp edge

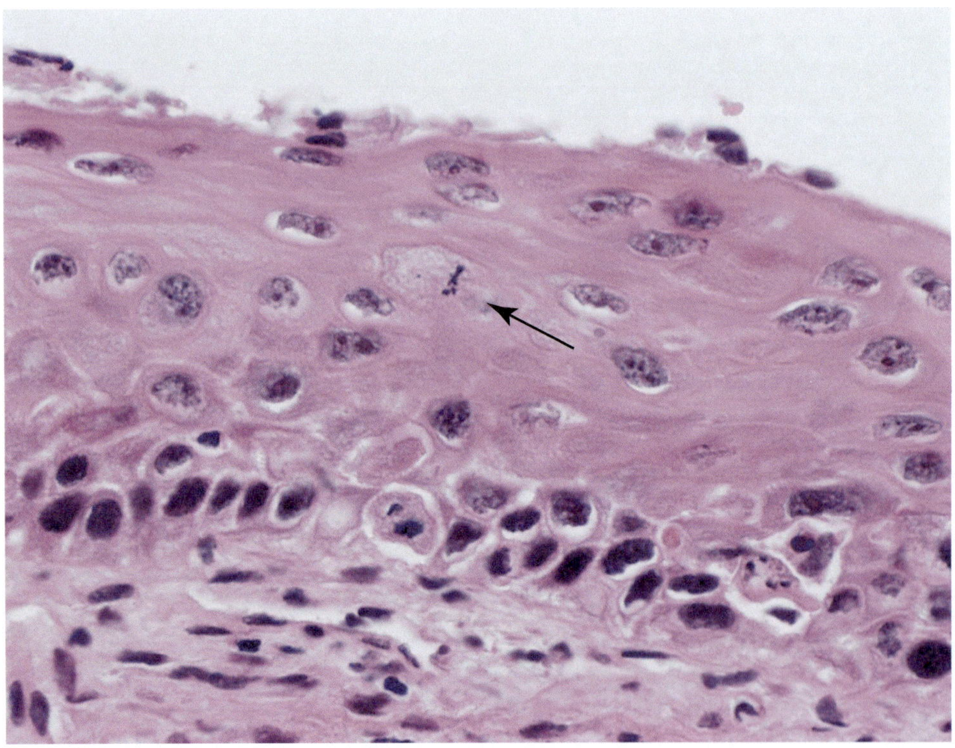

Fig. 1.3 HSIL (CIN 2) mimicking LSIL with nuclear abnormalities, even though confined to the lower third, showing significant nuclear hyperchromasia, irregular nuclear sizes and shapes, and mitotic activity in the middle third (arrow), which justified an HSIL diagnosis

HPV, as represented by the "one virus, one lesion" concept [18]. Therefore, women with an LSIL diagnosis are generally monitored.

1.1.2 HSIL

HSIL is a neoplastic condition resulting from the integration of high-risk HPV DNA, followed by uncontrolled E6 and E7 expression, which inactivates *TP53* and *RB*, respectively. As mentioned above, its morphologic spectrum includes CIN 2 and CIN 3, with a significant risk of the coexistence or development of invasive carcinoma.

HSIL incidence increases significantly around 30s, and in general, there are no clinical manifestations. HSIL is most often detected on biopsy taken from women who were referred for colposcopy because of positive cervical smear results. In cases of genital bleeding or the existence of colposcopically visible lesions, the coexistence of invasive carcinoma should be a concern. Another scenario in routine settings is an association with adenocarcinoma in situ or invasive adenocarcinoma.

Microscopically, HSIL is characterized by an expansion of the basal cell population, which shows nuclear enlargement and overlapping, irregularity in nuclear size, and abnormal mitotic figures. Traditionally, HSIL is divided into CIN 2 (Fig. 1.4) and CIN 3 (Fig. 1.5) based on whether the extent of nuclear abnormalities is confined to the lower two thirds or extends to the upper third of the epithelium. Koilocytosis may be seen in cases with surface differentiation, and occasionally HSIL show significant surface maturation with hyperkeratosis and a granular layer (keratinizing HSIL) (Fig. 1.6). Some HSILs appear homogeneous and bear a close resemblance to immature squamous metaplasia, while others may be very pleomorphic. A subset of HSIL is thin, mimicking atrophy (thin HSIL) (Fig. 1.7). The WHO classification (2014) describes papillary SCC in situ as a variant of HSIL that shows papillary growth with fine fibrovascular stromal cores [15]. Such diagnoses should be made with a great caution and only after excluding stromal invasion on conization or hysterectomy specimens because of frequent coexistence of invasive foci [19].

The differential diagnosis of HSIL includes immature squamous metaplasia, atrophy, LSIL, and SCC with expans-

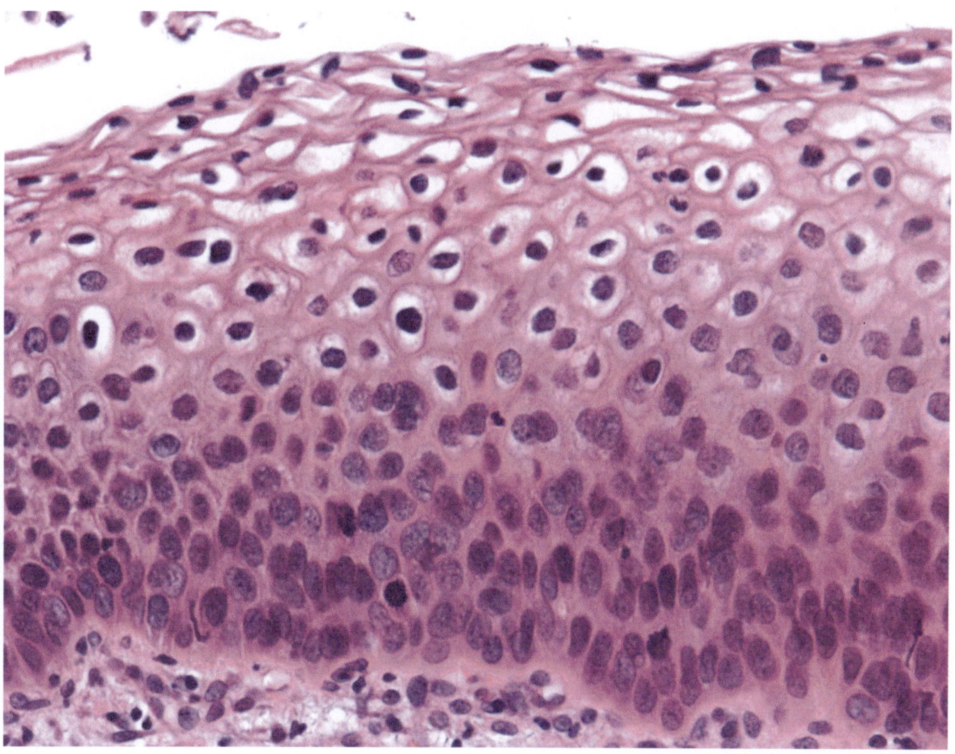

Fig. 1.4 HSIL (CIN 2) extending into the middle third of the layers with classical features and characterized by nuclear heterogeneous nuclear sizes and shapes

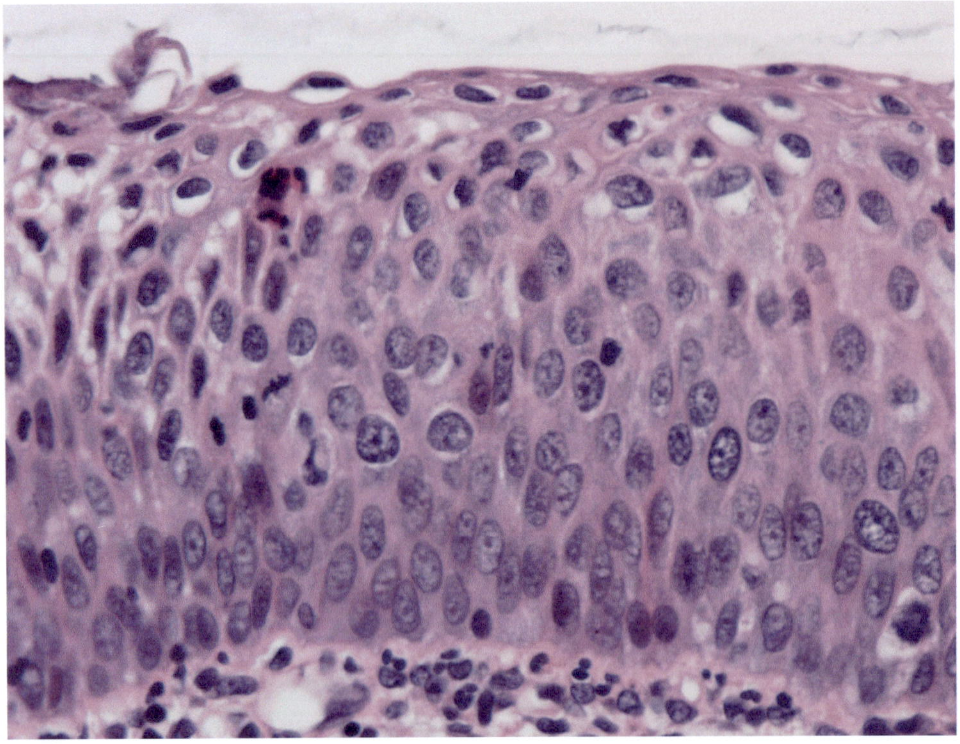

Fig. 1.5 HSIL (CIN 3), showing nuclear abnormalities with minimal surface maturation in the upper third of epithelium

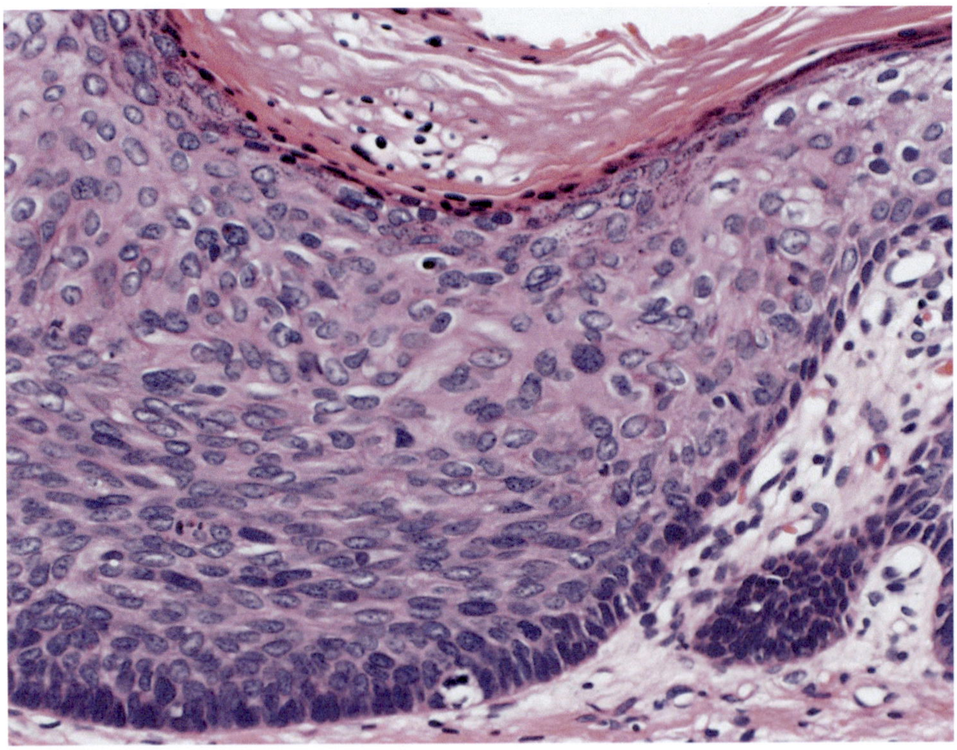

Fig. 1.6 Keratinizing HSIL (CIN 3), characterized by surface hyperkeratosis and parakeratosis

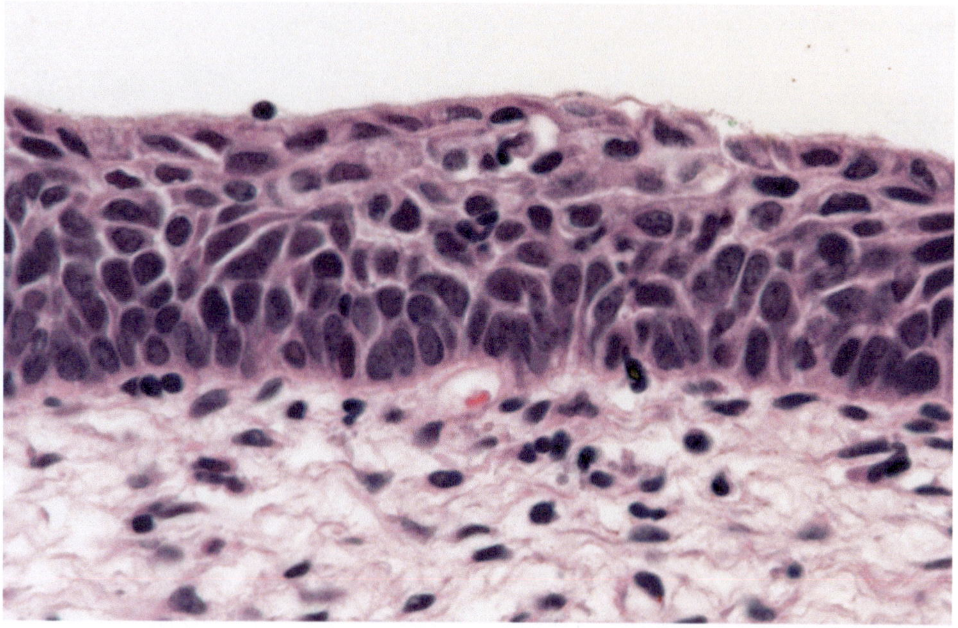

Fig. 1.7 Atrophic HSIL (CIN 3), showing less than ten cells in thickness

ile invasion. Significant nuclear abnormalities suggest an HSIL diagnosis, while bland nuclear morphology imparts a close resemblance to immature metaplasia. This problem can be solved by subsequent tests. Immunohistochemically HSIL shows diffuse and strong ("block-positive") nuclear and cytoplasmic staining for p16^{INK4a}, while immature squamous metaplasia and atrophy are negative or only show weak or focal staining. Atypical immature metaplasia, representing LSIL or immature condyloma, may also be positive for p16^{INK4a} and, thus, can be problematic. In such situations, the addition of Ki-67 IHC is recommended, where in HSIL cases the labeling index increases up to 50%.

1.1.3 Condyloma Acuminatum

Condyloma acuminatum is a benign papillary proliferation of the squamous epithelium, due to low-risk HPV infection, such as types 6 and 11. As mentioned previously, it is regarded as LSIL, but should be distinguished from flat LSIL ("flat condyloma"), which is mostly due to high-risk HPV infections. Microscopically, these lesions are composed of stratified squamous epithelium covering fibrovascular stroma, which forms a knuckle-like papillary proliferation. The epithelium may be thickened and shows koilocytosis, but these prototypical features are rather uncommon in cases of cervix in contrast to vulvar cases. Moreover, the epithelium is generally composed of immature-looking cells without prototypical koilocytosis and is designated as "immature papillary squamous metaplasia," which should be distinguished from HSIL or papillary SCC.

1.2 Biomarkers for SIL

There are a variety of biomarkers available to aid histologic and cytologic interpretations. Such ancillary methods include Ki-67, p16^{INK4a}, ProEX (MCM2/TOP2 double-staining kit), CINtec® PLUS (16^{INK4a}/Ki-67 double-staining kit), MN protein, L1 protein, p63/p73, cyclin, telomerase, c-myc mRNA, PIK3CA, HPV E6/E7 mRNA, aneuploidy, and DNA methylation. Among these Ki-67 and p16^{INK4a} IHC is widely used in routine histopathologic practice.

Ki-67 is a proliferation antigen expressed during the G1, S, and G2/M phases of the cell cycle and, thus, reflects proliferation. A normal stratified squamous epithelium has proliferation zone in the parabasal layer rather than in the basal layer. Conversely, intraepithelial neoplasia shows an expansion of basal layer composed of cells positive for Ki-67. However, in cases of reactive atypia or transient HPV infection, basal cells can be positive for Ki-67, necessitating a combination of morphologic assessment and

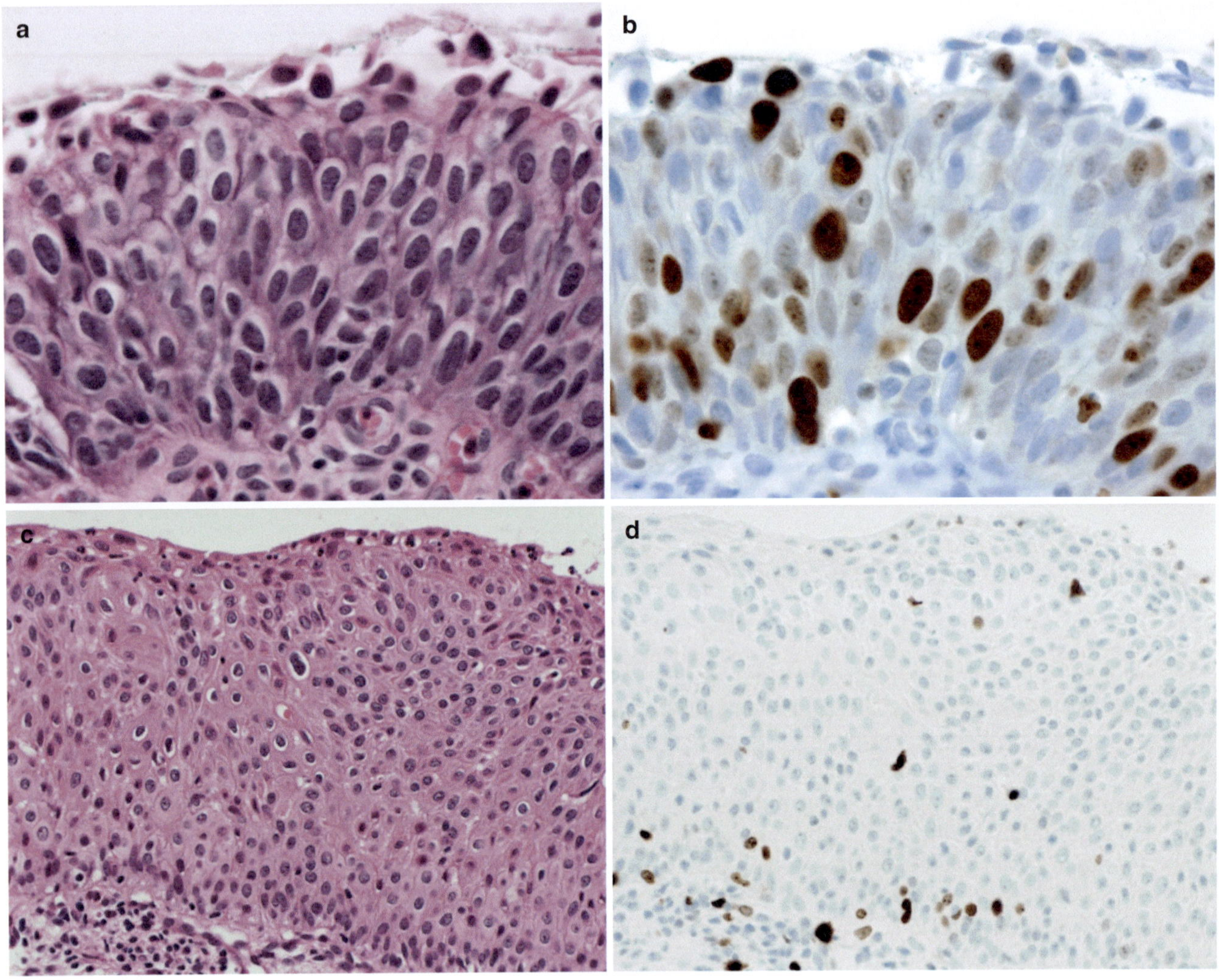

Fig. 1.8 Ki-67 immunohistochemistry. HSIL (CIN 3) (**a**), showing Ki-67-positive cells in the full thickness of the epithelium (**b**), and immature metaplasia (**c**), showing only scattered Ki-67-positive cells (**d**)

Ki-67 IHC for correct diagnosis [20]. A normal stratified squamous epithelium has a Ki-67 labeling index of less than 10%, while an index exceeding 20% or 5% in basal or middle third layers, respectively, or the existence of any Ki-67-positive cells in the upper third layer is indicative of the diagnosis of CIN (Fig. 1.8a, b) [20]. Immature squamous metaplasia only shows occasional Ki-67-positive cells (Fig. 1.8c, d), but it should be kept in mind that during the secretory phase, there is a transient elevation of the Ki-67 labeling index [21].

The p16^{INK4a} is a cyclin-dependent kinase inhibitor involved in cell cycle regulation that is encoded by the tumor suppressor gene *CDKN2A* (*P16INK4A*). Subsequent to HPV infection, p16^{INK4a} is overexpressed as a consequence of the loss of a negative feedback loop that results from the inactivation of RB by the viral oncoprotein E7. Therefore, it is regarded as a surrogate biomarker that indicates neoplastic transformation caused by the integration of HPV DNA; p16^{INK4a} overexpression suggests an HSIL diagnosis [22, 23]. p16^{INK4a} IHC should only be regarded as positive in cases of diffuse and strong ("block positive") staining. Furthermore, HSIL may show a gradation in the upper portion of the epithelium in cases of surface maturation (Fig. 1.9a, b). When HSIL is a diagnostic concern, the negative p16^{INK4a} staining suggests alternative diagnoses including atypical immature metaplasia or atrophy (Fig. 1.9c, d). p16^{INK4a} IHC results

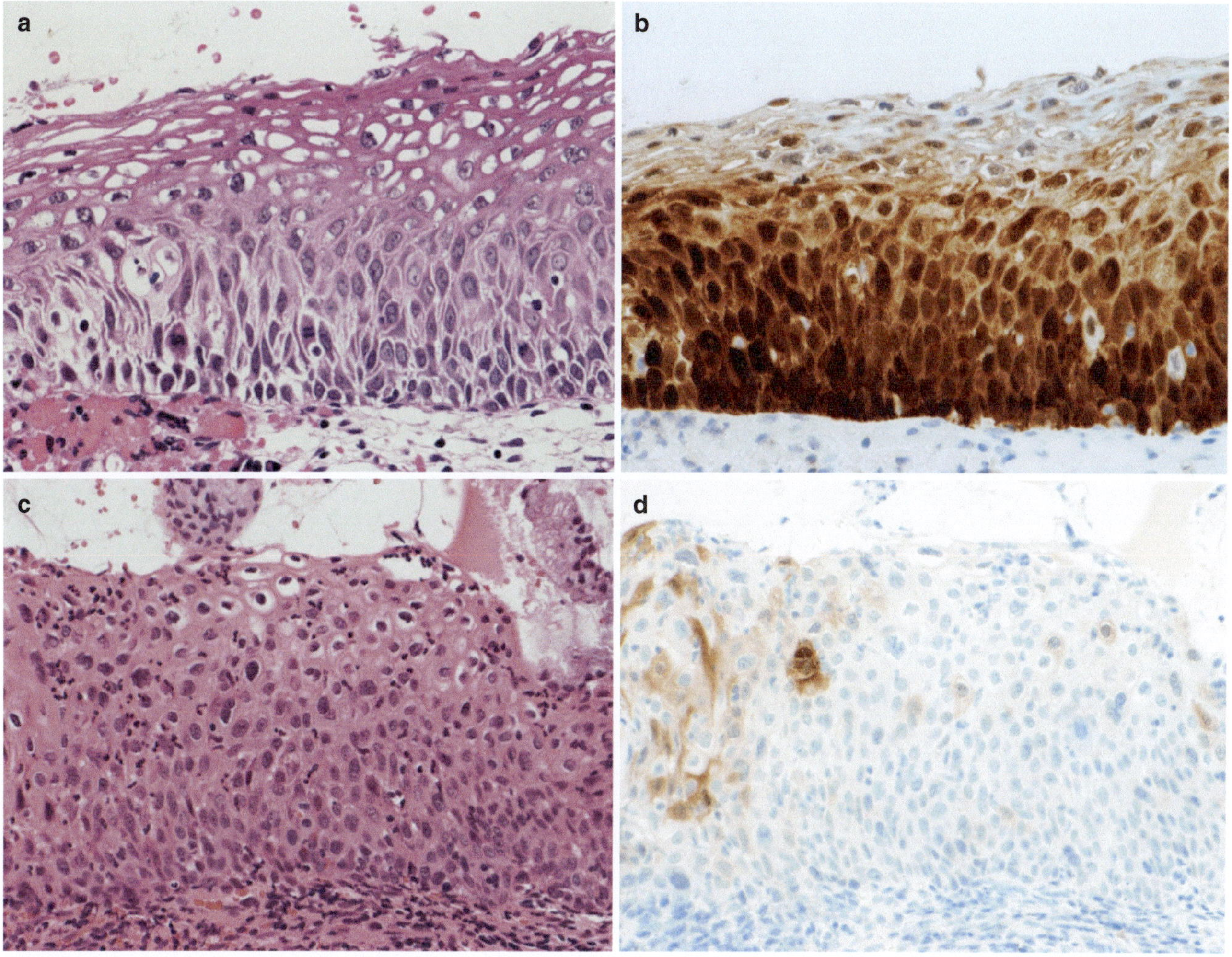

Fig. 1.9 p16^{INK4a} immunohistochemistry. HSIL (CIN 1) (**a**) showing p16^{INK4a} immunoreactivity in the lower two thirds, with gradation in the upper portion (**b**). LSIL with metaplastic features (atypical immature metaplasia) (**c**). Metaplastic epithelium with mildly enlarged nuclei showing focal and weak p16^{INK4a} immunoreactivity (**d**)

should also be combined with morphology, as approximately 30% of LSILs are also positive for p16^{INK4a}.

The LAST guideline recommends using p16^{INK4a} IHC in situations when (1) a distinction between HSIL/CIN 3 and immature metaplasia or atrophy is difficult, (2) there is a suspicion of HSIL/CIN 2, (3) there are discrepant opinions among pathologists regarding the diagnosis, and (4) there is negative or an apparent LSIL case with a cytological interpretation of ASC-H or HSIL [10]. The 4th is considered to be an indication for quality assurance.

Combining Ki-67 and p16^{INK4a} IHC can increase the sensitivity and specificity of SIL diagnoses (Fig. 1.10a–c). The significance of p16^{INK4a} expression in LSIL cases is an intriguing issue, as it has been suggested that p16^{INK4a}-positive LSIL may progress to HSIL more frequently than previously appreciated [24, 25].

Antibodies raised against the HPV capsid protein L1 for IHC and cocktails of probes recognizing HPV for ISH are commercially available and can be used to label abnormal nuclei that do not fit with typical koilocytosis in questionable cases (Fig. 1.11a, b). In addition to determining the presence or absence of HPV, ISH can distinguish between productive and transforming infections. The former is suggested by a diffuse signal pattern, and the latter by a dot-like pattern that indicates integration of HPV DNA into the host genome (Fig. 1.12a, b).

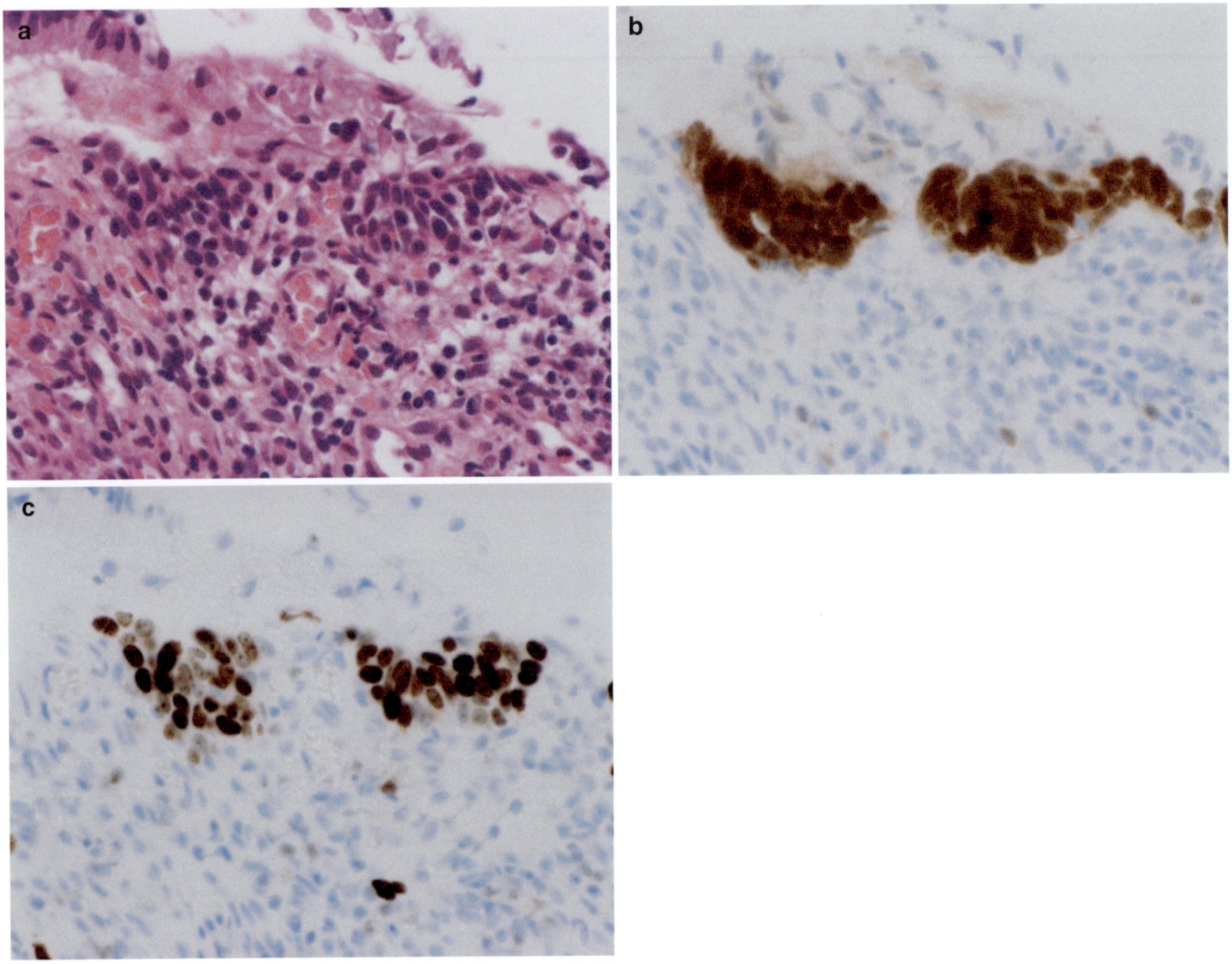

Fig. 1.10 16^{INK4a} and Ki-67 immunohistochemistry. A thin and tiny focus of atypical cells (**a**), showing diffuse and strong ("block-positive") immunoreactivity (**b**), and a significant increase in Ki-67-positive cells (**c**), confirming the diagnosis of HSIL (CIN 3)

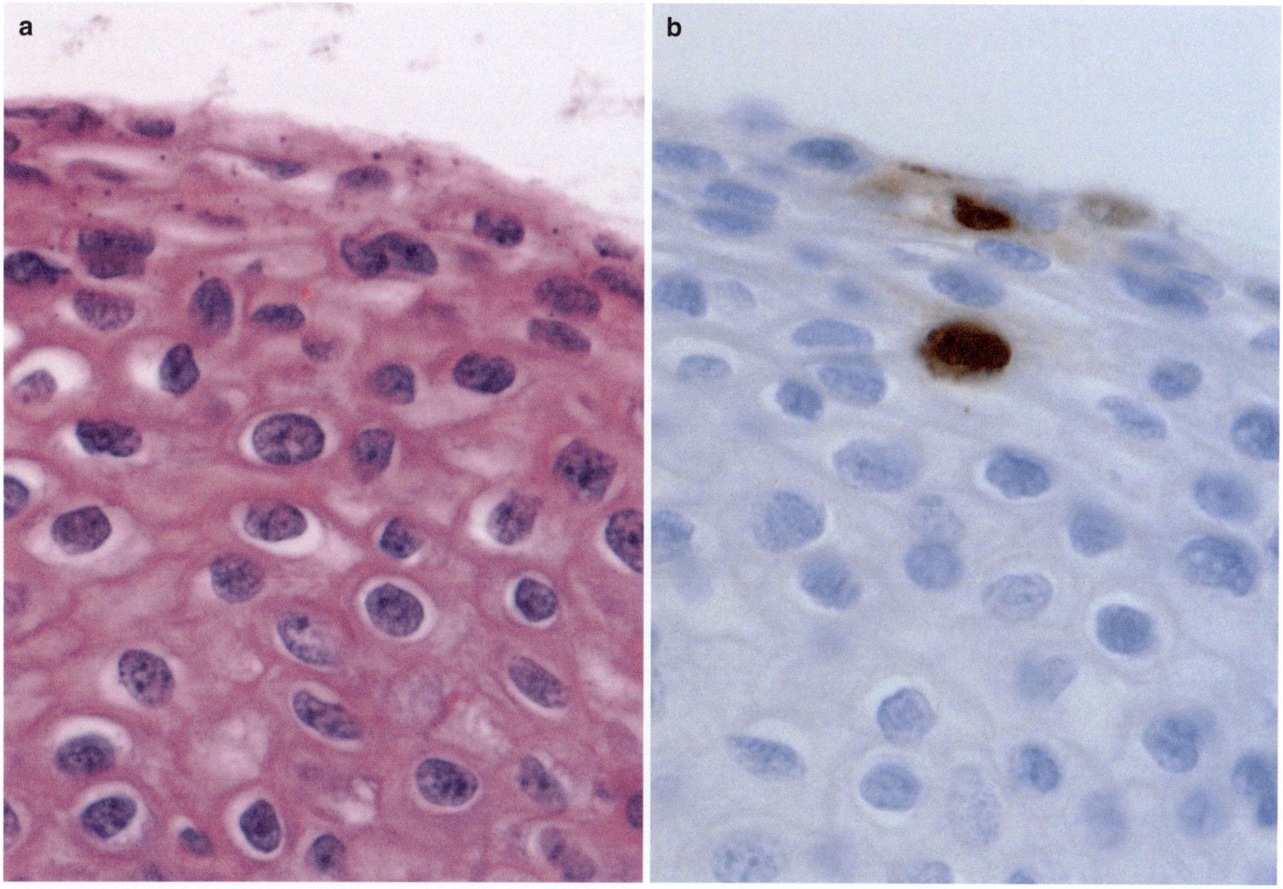

Fig. 1.11 HPV capsid L1 immunohistochemistry employing a monoclonal antibody against capsid L1, which recognizes HPV types 6, 11, 14, 18, 31, 42, 51, 52, 56, and 58 (Clone K1H8; DAKO, Glostrup, Denmark). A subset of superficial cells with mild nuclear enlargement and perinuclear clearing that do not best fit with prototypical koilocytosis (**a**), showing positive nuclear L1 staining (**b**). Microscopically it was difficult to diagnose the lesion as an HPV infection

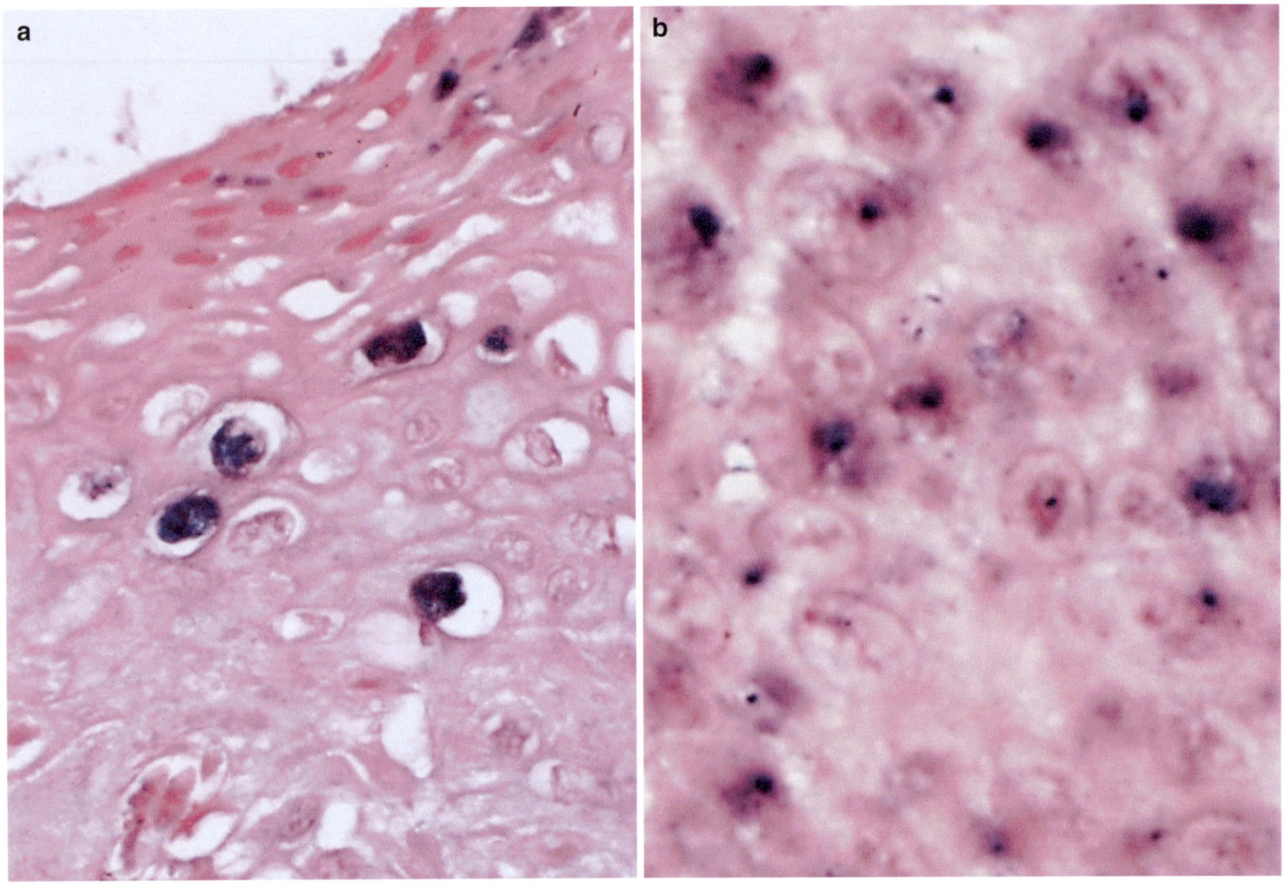

Fig. 1.12 HPV in situ hybridization, employing a cocktail of labeled HPV genomic probes, i.e., INFORM® HPV III Family 16 probe (**b**), which recognizes HPV types 16, 18, 31, 33, 35, 39, 45, 51, 52, 56, 58, and 66. Superficial and intermediate cells in an LSIL case with nuclei showing a diffuse pattern of labeling, which indicates a productive infection (**a**), whereas HSIL shows atypical cells with a dot pattern as a result of the HPV DNA integration into the host genome (transforming infection) (**b**)

References

1. Rubin IC. The pathological diagnosis of incipient carcinoma of the uterus. Am J Obstet. 1910;62:668–76.
2. Broders AC. Carcinoma in situ contrasted with benign penetrating epithelium. JAMA. 1932;99:1670–4.
3. Reagan JW, Seidemann IL, Saracusa Y. The cellular morphology of carcinoma in situ and dysplasia or atypical hyperplasia of the uterine cervix. Cancer. 1953;6(2):224–34.
4. Richart RM, Barron BA. A follow-up study of patients with cervical dysplasia. Am J Obstet Gynecol. 1969;105(3):386–93.
5. Durst M, Gissmann L, Ikenberg H, zur Hausen H. A papillomavirus DNA from a cervical carcinoma and its prevalence in cancer biopsy samples from different geographic regions. Proc Natl Acad Sci U S A. 1983;80(12):3812–5.
6. Gissmann L, Wolnik L, Ikenberg H, Koldovsky U, Schnurch HG, zur Hausen H. Human papillomavirus types 6 and 11 DNA sequences in genital and laryngeal papillomas and in some cervical cancers. Proc Natl Acad Sci U S A. 1983;80(2):560–3.
7. Crum CP, Ikenberg H, Richart RM, Gissman L. Human papillomavirus type 16 and early cervical neoplasia. N Engl J Med. 1984;310(14):880–3. https://doi.org/10.1056/NEJM198404053101403.
8. Winkler B, Crum CP, Fujii T, Ferenczy A, Boon M, Braun L, Lancaster WD, Richart RM. Koilocytotic lesions of the cervix. The relationship of mitotic abnormalities to the presence of papillomavirus antigens and nuclear DNA content. Cancer. 1984;53(5):1081–7.
9. The 1988 Bethesda system for reporting cervical/vaginal cytologic diagnoses. Developed and approved at a National Cancer Institute workshop, Bethesda, Maryland, USA, December 12-13, 1988. J Reprod Med. 1989;34(10):779–85.
10. Darragh TM, Colgan TJ, Thomas Cox J, Heller DS, Henry MR, Luff RD, McCalmont T, Nayar R, Palefsky JM, Stoler MH, Wilkinson EJ, Zaino RJ, Wilbur DC, Members of the LPWG. The lower Anogenital squamous terminology standardization project for HPV-associated lesions: background and consensus recommendations from the College of American Pathologists and the American Society for Colposcopy and Cervical Pathology. Int J Gynecol Pathol. 2013;32(1):76–115. https://doi.org/10.1097/PGP.0b013e31826916c7.
11. Kurman RJ, International Agency for Research on Cancer, World Health Organization. WHO classification of tumours of female reproductive organs. World Health Organization classification of tumours. 4th ed. Lyon: International Agency for Research on Cancer; 2014.
12. Gage JC, Schiffman M, Hunt WC, Joste N, Ghosh A, Wentzensen N, Wheeler CM, New Mexico HPVPRSC. Cervical histopathol-

ogy variability among laboratories: a population-based statewide investigation. Am J Clin Pathol. 2013;139(3):330–5. https://doi.org/10.1309/AJCPSD3ZXJXP7NNB.
13. Dalla Palma P, Giorgi Rossi P, Collina G, Buccoliero AM, Ghiringhello B, Gilioli E, Onnis GL, Aldovini D, Galanti G, Casadei G, Aldi M, Gomes VV, Giubilato P, Ronco G, Group NP. The reproducibility of CIN diagnoses among different pathologists: data from histology reviews from a multicenter randomized study. Am J Clin Pathol. 2009;132(1):125–32. https://doi.org/10.1309/AJCPBRK7D1YIUWFP.
14. Wright TC Jr, Massad LS, Dunton CJ, Spitzer M, Wilkinson EJ, Solomon D, American Society for Colposcopy and Cervical Pathology-Sponsored Consensus Conference. 2006 consensus guidelines for the management of women with cervical intraepithelial neoplasia or adenocarcinoma in situ. Am J Obstet Gynecol. 2007;197(4):340–5. https://doi.org/10.1016/j.ajog.2007.07.050.
15. Stoler M, Bergeron C, Colgan TJ, Ferenczy AS, Herrington CS, Kim KR, Loening T, Schneider A, Sherman ME, Wilbur DC, Wright T. Squamous cell tumors and precursors. In: Kurman RJ, Carcangiu ML, Herrington CS, Young RH, editors. WHO classification of tumours of female reproductive organs. Lyon: IARC; 2014.
16. Darragh TM, Colgan TJ, Cox JT, Heller DS, Henry MR, Luff RD, McCalmont T, Nayar R, Palefsky JM, Stoler MH, Wilkinson EJ, Zaino RJ, Wilbur DC, Members of LPWG. The lower Anogenital squamous terminology standardization project for HPV-associated lesions: background and consensus recommendations from the College of American Pathologists and the American Society for Colposcopy and Cervical Pathology. J Low Genit Tract Dis. 2012;16(3):205–42. https://doi.org/10.1097/LGT.0b013e31825c31dd.
17. Cho NH, Kang S, Hong S, Jeong GB, Choi IW, Choi HJ, Choi HK. Multinucleation of koilocytes is in fact multilobation and is related to aberration of the G2 checkpoint. J Clin Pathol. 2005;58(6):576–82. https://doi.org/10.1136/jcp.2004.022152.
18. Quint W, Jenkins D, Molijn A, Struijk L, van de Sandt M, Doorbar J, Mols J, Van Hoof C, Hardt K, Struyf F, Colau B. One virus, one lesion—individual components of CIN lesions contain a specific HPV type. J Pathol. 2012;227(1):62–71. https://doi.org/10.1002/path.3970.
19. Nagura M, Koshiyama M, Matsumura N, Kido A, Baba T, Abiko K, Hamanishi J, Yamaguchi K, Mikami Y, Konishi I. Clinical approaches to treating papillary squamous cell carcinoma of the uterine cervix. BMC Cancer. 2014;14:784. https://doi.org/10.1186/1471-2407-14-784.
20. Mittal K. Utility of proliferation-associated marker MIB-1 in evaluating lesions of the uterine cervix. Adv Anat Pathol. 1999;6(4):177–85.
21. Konishi I, Fujii S, Nonogaki H, Nanbu Y, Iwai T, Mori T. Immunohistochemical analysis of estrogen receptors, progesterone receptors, Ki-67 antigen, and human papillomavirus DNA in normal and neoplastic epithelium of the uterine cervix. Cancer. 1991;68(6):1340–50.
22. Kalof AN, Evans MF, Simmons-Arnold L, Beatty BG, Cooper K. p16INK4A immunoexpression and HPV in situ hybridization signal patterns: potential markers of high-grade cervical intraepithelial neoplasia. Am J Surg Pathol. 2005;29(5):674–9. doi: 00000478-200505000-00015 [pii].
23. Klaes R, Friedrich T, Spitkovsky D, Ridder R, Rudy W, Petry U, Dallenbach-Hellweg G, Schmidt D, von Knebel Doeberitz M. Overexpression of p16(INK4A) as a specific marker for dysplastic and neoplastic epithelial cells of the cervix uteri. Int J Cancer. 2001;92(2):276–84. https://doi.org/10.1002/ijc.1174. [pii].
24. Wang JL, Zheng BY, Li XD, Angstrom T, Lindstrom MS, Wallin KL. Predictive significance of the alterations of p16INK4A, p14ARF, p53, and proliferating cell nuclear antigen expression in the progression of cervical cancer. Clin Cancer Res. 2004;10(7):2407–14.
25. Queiroz C, Silva TC, Alves VA, Villa LL, Costa MC, Travassos AG, Filho JB, Studart E, Cheto T, de Freitas LA. P16(INK4a) expression as a potential prognostic marker in cervical pre-neoplastic and neoplastic lesions. Pathol Res Pract. 2006;202(2):77–83. doi:S0344-0338(05)00216-5 [pii]. https://doi.org/10.1016/j.prp.2005.08.012.

Adenocarcinoma and Its Precursor of the Uterine Cervix: Current Concept

2

Suzuko Moritani

Abstract

Cervical adenocarcinoma accounts for up to 25% of all cervical carcinomas. Adenocarcinoma in situ (AIS) is a widely recognized precursor of adenocarcinoma. While most cervical adenocarcinomas are associated with high-risk human papillomavirus (HPV), the minority are HPV-negative. The most common cervical adenocarcinoma is endocervical adenocarcinoma, usual type, which is characterized by mucin-poor neoplastic cells. Classification of mucinous carcinoma has markedly changed. Gastric-type mucinous carcinoma is a recently recognized subtype that includes minimal deviation adenocarcinoma as the extremely well-differentiated end of this category. It is HPV-negative and clinically aggressive. Endometrioid carcinoma is a poorly defined subtype, and differential diagnosis from endocervical adenocarcinoma, usual type, is subjective. Endometrioid carcinoma is considered to be rare, and its incidence is estimated to be less than 5%. In recent years, most cases of clear cell carcinoma have not been associated with diethylstilbestrol (DES) exposure. Serous carcinoma of the cervix is extremely rare, and metastatic carcinoma should be excluded before its diagnosis. Mesonephric carcinoma is not associated with high-risk HPV.

Keywords

AIS · HPV · Usual type · Gastric type · p16 · SMILE · Villoglandular carcinoma · Pseudoneoplastic glandular lesion · Mesonephric carcinoma

S. Moritani
Division of Diagnostic Pathology, Shiga University of Medical Science, Ohtsu, Shiga, Japan
e-mail: mori@belle.shiga-med.ac.jp

2.1 General

There has been growing attention to glandular lesions of the uterine cervix during the past several decades with the increased incidence of cervical adenocarcinoma. Recently identified immunohistochemical markers and advanced genetic research have brought new insights to its etiology and histological classification relevant to clinical practice.

Adenocarcinoma now accounts for approximately 25% of all cervical carcinomas. More than 90% of cervical glandular neoplasms are related to high-risk HPV infection. HPV16, 18, and 45 are the common types [1, 2]. A subset of rare histological types are known to occur without HPV infection and have distinct clinicopathological features.

The most recent World Health Organization (WHO) classification of cervical glandular lesions is shown in Table 2.1 [3].

Table 2.1 Cervical glandular tumors and precursors

Adenocarcinoma in situ
Adenocarcinoma
Endocervical adenocarcinoma, usual type
Mucinous carcinoma, NOS
Gastric type
Intestinal type
Signet-ring cell type
Villoglandular carcinoma
Endometrioid carcinoma
Clear cell carcinoma
Serous carcinoma
Mesonephric carcinoma
Adenocarcinoma admixed with neuroendocrine carcinoma

T. Moriya (ed.), *Pathology of Female Cancers*, https://doi.org/10.1007/978-981-10-8606-9_2

2.2 Precursor of Cervical Adenocarcinoma

Adenocarcinoma in situ (AIS) is the undisputed precursor of cervical adenocarcinoma [4–6]. Preinvasive cervical glandular neoplasms less atypical than AIS conceptually exist, and such lesions have been called "glandular dysplasia" or "cervical glandular intraepithelial neoplasia" [5, 7]. Although there have been attempts to diagnose glandular lesions less atypical than AIS with objective scoring system [8], interobserver reproducibility of its diagnosis is practically lacking. The biological and clinical significance of glandular dysplasia remains controversial [9–11]. Some investigators believe that glandular dysplasia could be classified either as reactive atypia or the lower end of AIS. Consequently, glandular dysplasia was excluded from the most recent WHO classification [3].

2.2.1 Clinical Features of AIS

AIS typically occurs in patients in their 30 or 40 years, being 10–15 years earlier than invasive adenocarcinoma [12]. Patients are usually asymptomatic, and cervical cytology is the most frequent detection modality. As there is no visible gross abnormality, the lesion is not detected by radiological images or colposcopy.

2.2.2 Histological Findings of AIS

AIS typically arises in the transformation zone as well as squamous intraepithelial lesions. Neoplastic epithelial cells proliferate along the surface epithelium and endocervical glands and replace normal glandular epithelial cells. The overall architecture of native endocervical glands is well preserved and there is no or minimal stromal reaction. There is usually a sharp demarcation between neoplastic and nonneoplastic epithelial cells (Fig. 2.1a, b). The extent of neoplastic involvement could be very subtle [13] to wide, and neoplastic cells involve both surface and deeper portions of the glands. Some lesions extend up to 30 mm in the cervical canal [14]. Multicentric lesions are seen in 10–15% of cases. Coexistent squamous intraepithelial lesions (SIL) are not rare [15, 16]. AIS may be found incidentally in the course of examination or treatment of SIL.

Neoplastic cells have enlarged hyperchromatic nuclei. The nuclei show various degrees of stratification. Mitosis and apoptosis are typically increased [8, 17] (Fig. 2.1a). Neoplastic epithelial cells are occasionally piled up and form papillary protrusion, bridging, and cribriform structures (Fig. 2.1c). The cribriform structure of AIS should be limited to a single gland lumen and should not be fused with adjacent neoplastic glands. Complete obstruction of the glandular lumen by solid proliferation is also observed. AIS may involve various types of hyperplastic lesions (Fig. 2.1d) and tunnel clusters.

There are several histological subtypes of AIS classified by cytological features of neoplastic cells. These subtypes frequently coexist within the same lesion. The subtypes are not clinically significant; however, it is useful for pathologists to recognize cytological features of different subtypes as AIS. The most common subtype is the endocervical or "usual" type (Fig. 2.1a). It is characterized by eosinophilic cytoplasm resembling normal endocervical glands. Small amounts of intracytoplasmic mucin are usually observed. The intestinal type is also relatively common and characterized by goblet cells (Fig. 2.1e). Due to abundant intracytoplasmic mucin, nuclear atypia and stratification appear less prominent than in other subtypes. The endometrioid type resembles the usual type; however, neoplastic cells have no visible intracytoplasmic mucin. Nuclear stratification is also more prominent than in the usual type. The adenosquamous type consists of mixed neoplastic cells showing both squamous and glandular differentiation. The adenosquamous type must be distinguished from AIS coexistent with SIL. In the latter lesion, AIS and SIL have discrete areas. Stratified mucin-producing intraepithelial lesion (SMILE) is an intraepithelial neoplasm resembling high-grade squamous intraepithelial lesion (HSIL) with scattered mucin-containing cells [18] (Fig. 2.1f). Differences between SMILE and AIS of adenosquamous type remain unclear, and some consider SMILE to be a form of adenosquamous CIS. Other rare subtypes of AIS have been reported including tubal [19], gastric [20], villoglandular, serous, and clear cell AIS.

2.2.3 Immunohistochemical Findings of AIS

Most cases, except for those with rare non-HPV-related subtypes, show diffuse and strong p16 expression in both nuclei and cytoplasm (Fig. 2.1b). Overall positivity of general proliferation marker, Ki-67, is significantly increased. ProExC is a marker of high-risk HPV-related cell proliferation and increased number of positive cells is seen in AIS [21, 22]. Estrogen receptor (ER) and progesterone receptor (PgR) expression is typically negative. Bcl-2 is negative or only weakly positive [23].

2.2.4 Differential Diagnosis of AIS

Reactive/reparative atypia can show prominent nuclear enlargement and visible nucleoli. However, the degree of nuclear stratification and frequency of mitosis and apoptosis are significantly lower than in AIS. Background inflammation is usually evident.

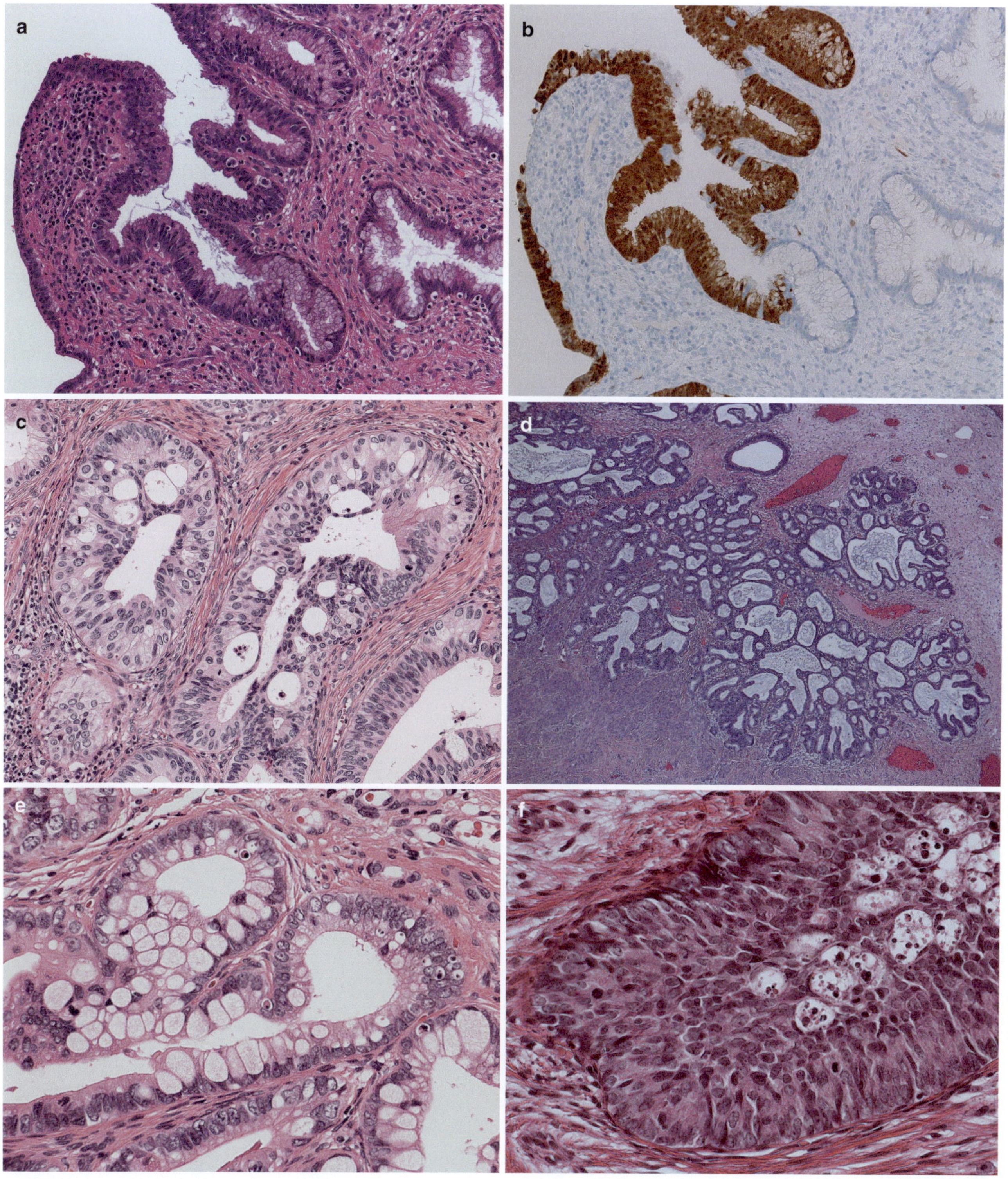

Fig. 2.1 Adenocarcinoma in situ (AIS). (**a**) AIS of usual type. (**b**) p16 is strongly positive in AIS. (**c**) Cribriform pattern in AIS. (**d**) Florid AIS involving hyperplastic endocervical glands. (**e**) AIS of intestinal type. (**f**) SMILE

Tubal and tuboendometrial metaplasias and superficial endometriosis are the most difficult benign lesions to differentiate from AIS [24–26] (Fig. 2.3a). Although the presence of cilia in tubal and tuboendometrial metaplasia and endometrial stromal cells surrounding endometriosis is clue to these benign lesions, such features are not always apparent, and both show nuclear stratification, increased proliferative activity, and p16 expression. However, p16 expression is patchy with heterogenous signal intensity in contrast to diffuse and strong positivity in AIS. Bcl-2 expression is usually positive in tubal metaplasia, tuboendometrial metaplasia, and endometriosis [23, 27, 28] (Fig. 2.3b).

Intraepithelial extension of endometrial endometrioid adenocarcinoma closely mimics AIS. Endometrial endometrioid adenocarcinoma is positive for ER and PgR, whereas AIS is usually negative for these markers [29]. P16 expression is varied in endometrial endometrioid adenocarcinoma, but not diffuse and strongly positive as in AIS [30, 31].

2.3 Adenocarcinoma

The presence of stromal invasion is necessary for the diagnosis of cervical adenocarcinoma. The extent of stromal invasion varies from case to case, and the prognosis of cervical adenocarcinoma is largely dependent on its stage. Many attempts have been made to define early invasive or microinvasive adenocarcinoma, which has minimal risk of lymph node metastasis and recurrence. Some investigators have reported an upper limit of depth/thickness of early invasive adenocarcinoma ranging from 1 to 5 mm [32–36]. Others defined the upper limit of tumor volume (500 mm^3) [37]. Although the 2003 WHO classification of tumors [7] listed early invasive adenocarcinoma as a category of glandular tumors and precursors, the current classification has eliminated this category because early invasive adenocarcinoma is defined by TNM/FIGO stage. Early invasive adenocarcinoma is equivalent to stage IA adenocarcinoma (less than 5 mm in depth and less than 7 mm in horizontal spread) [3] (Fig. 2.2a).

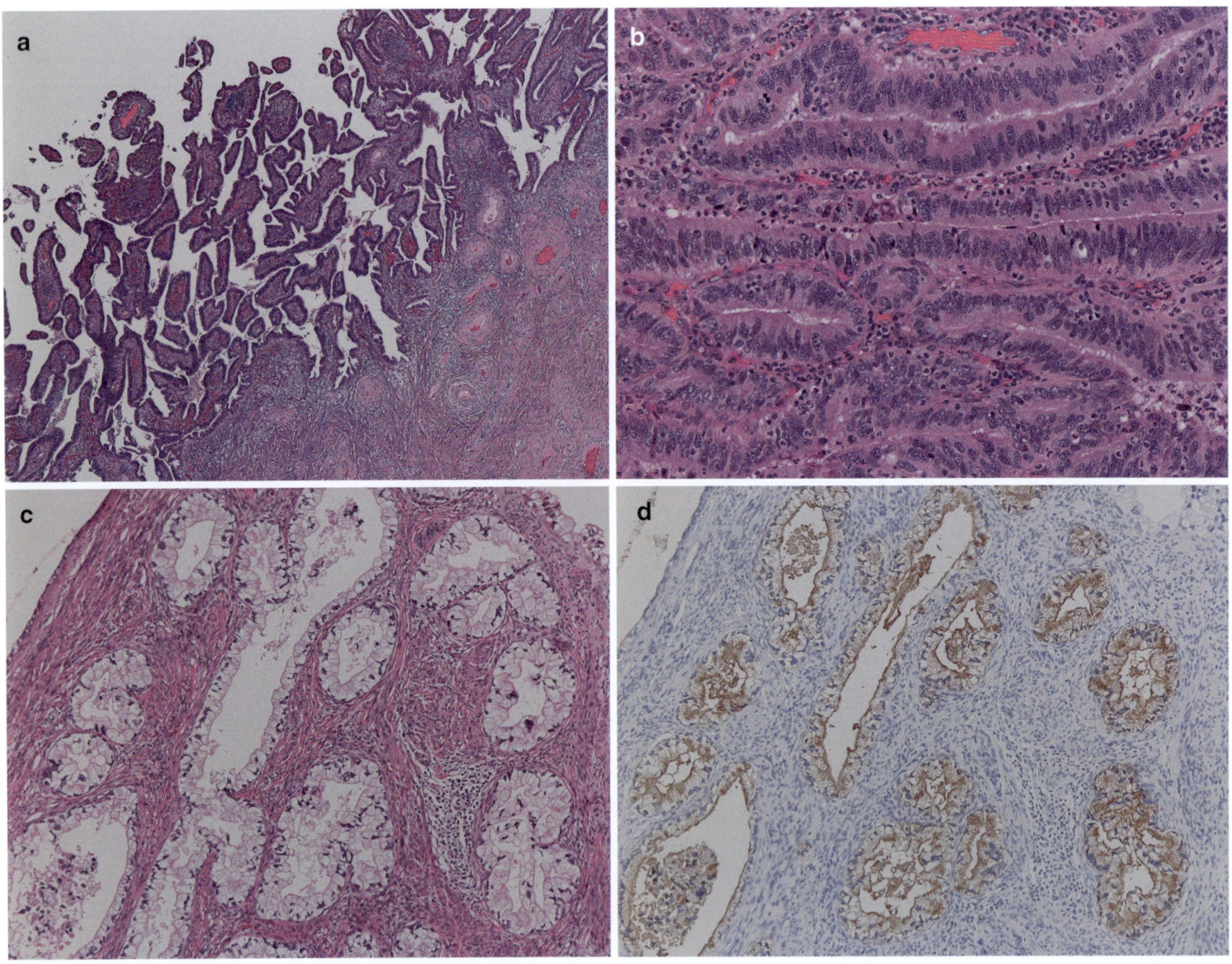

Fig. 2.2 Adenocarcinoma. (**a**) Early invasive adenocarcinoma (villoglandular carcinoma). (**b**) Endocervical adenocarcinoma, usual type. (**c**) Mucinous carcinoma, gastric type. (**d**) HIK-1083 expression in gastric-type mucinous carcinoma. (**e**) Endometrioid carcinoma. (**f**) Clear cell carcinoma. (**g**) Mesonephric carcinoma

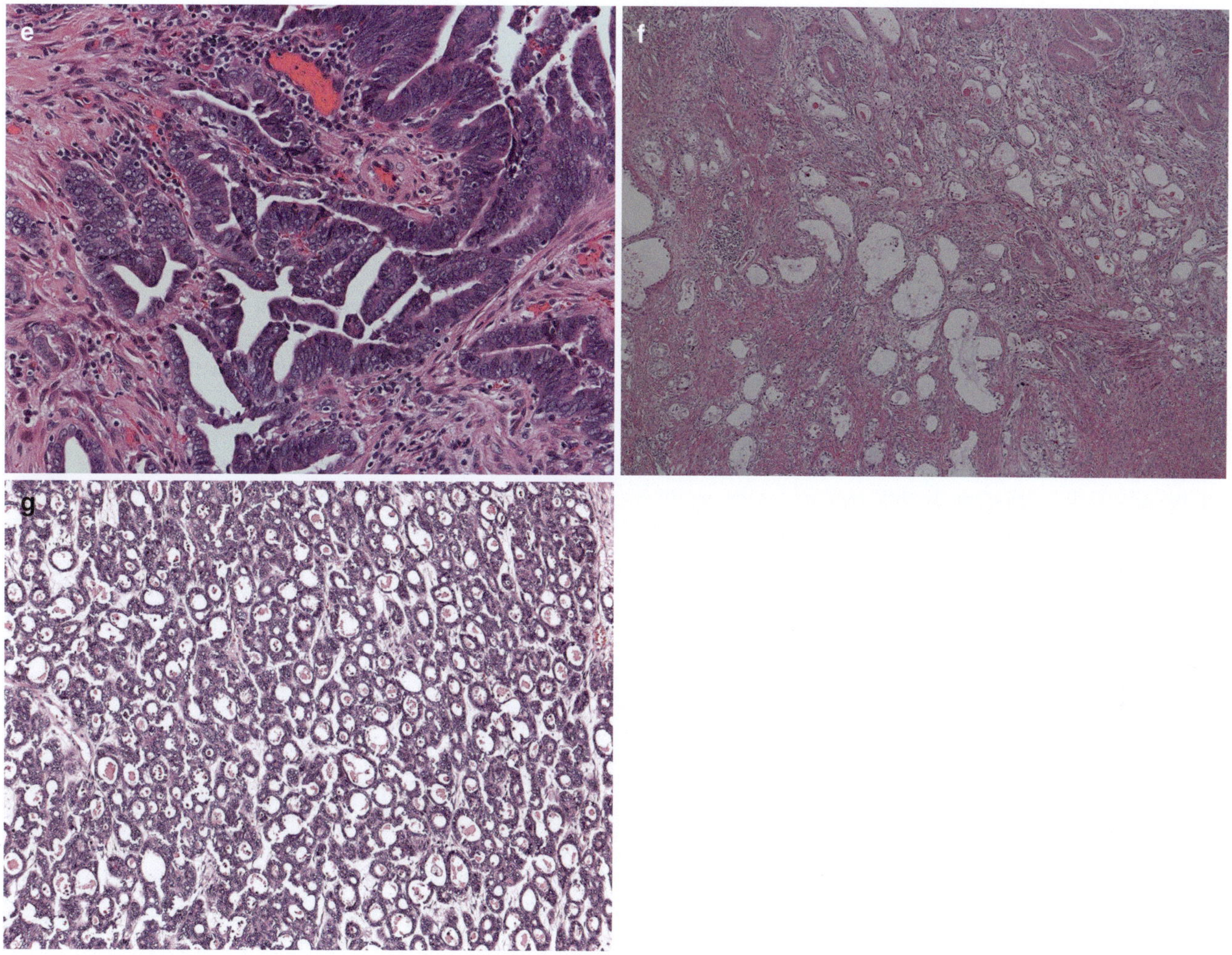

Fig. 2.2 (continued)

Cervical adenocarcinoma can be subclassified into high-risk HPV-associated and HPV-unassociated groups [38]. Most cervical adenocarcinomas are associated with high-risk HPV [1]. The HPV-unassociated group includes gastric-type mucinous carcinoma, clear cell carcinoma, and mesonephric carcinoma [39, 40]. Association with HPV remains controversial for endometrioid and serous carcinomas, whereas all other types are positive for HPV.

2.3.1 Clinical and Gross Features of Adenocarcinoma

The mean age of patients is approximately 50 years. Abnormal uterine bleeding is the most frequent symptom. Watery discharge is characteristic to gastric-type mucinous carcinoma. Grossly visible cervical abnormalities are seen in many cases. Tumors present exophytic, nodular, diffusely infiltrative, and ulcerative growth patterns. Diffusely infiltrative tumors show a characteristic barrel-shaped cervix.

2.3.2 Diagnostic Histological Features of Stromal Invasion

The earliest invasion is seen as finger-like projections of tumor cells from AIS into the stroma or scattered small clusters of free-floating tumor cells in the stroma. These tumor cells tend to have more abundant eosinophilic cytoplasm and larger nuclei than those of adjacent AIS. Desmoplastic stromal reaction and/or infiltration of chronic inflammatory cells is usually seen around invasive tumor cells. Distinction from extensive AIS, especially AIS involving hyperplastic endocervical glands, is difficult. The overall architecture of normal or hyperplastic endocervical glands is preserved in AIS (Fig. 2.1d), but not in invasive adenocarcinoma (Fig. 2.2a). Comparison of tumor contour to adjacent nonneoplastic glands may aid in this distinction. Invasive adenocarcinoma extends beyond the deepest endocervical glands. Close proximity of neoplastic glands to thick-walled blood vessels indicates stromal invasion. Typical invasive adenocarcinomas present prominent glandular crowding and complex architectural abnormalities with irregular branching, prominent papillary growth, confluence of the glands, and cribriform structures.

2.3.3 Histological Subtypes of Adenocarcinoma

2.3.3.1 Endocervical Adenocarcinoma, Usual Type

Endocervical adenocarcinoma, usual type, is the most common type, accounting for approximately 90% of all cervical adenocarcinomas. Most cases included in this category correspond to mucinous adenocarcinoma of endocervical type according to the former WHO classification. These tumors are usually well to moderately differentiated with papillary and cribriform patterns. Tumor cells are tall columnar-shaped and have eosinophilic to amphophilic cytoplasm (Fig. 2.2b). Intracytoplasmic mucin is relatively depleted but variably produced [41]. Nuclear pseudostratification is prominent and mitosis is increased. The apical situation of mitotic figures is characteristic ("floating mitotic figures"). Leukocytes are frequently seen in glandular lumens. The tumor is almost always HPV-related and diffusely positive for p16. Ki-67 and ProExC-positive cells are increased in number. ER and PgR expression is negative.

2.3.3.2 Mucinous Carcinoma

The tumor cells in mucinous carcinoma have prominent intracytoplasmic mucin.

Gastric-type mucinous carcinoma is a relatively newly defined concept with distinct clinicopathological features [20, 42]. It was classified as endocervical-type mucinous adenocarcinoma or minimal deviation adenocarcinoma (MDA) in the former WHO classification. MDA/adenoma malignum is currently regarded as an extremely well-differentiated form of gastric-type mucinous carcinoma. Gastric-type mucinous carcinoma comprises approximately 20–25% of all cervical adenocarcinomas [42]. Patients often present watery or mucoid discharge. It is not associated with high-risk HPV infection in its tumorigenesis [40, 43]. Lobular endocervical glandular hyperplasia (LEGH) and AIS of gastric type are potential precursor lesions [44]. Some cases are related to Peutz-Jeghers syndrome [20]. Gastric-type mucinous carcinoma is clinically aggressive compared to other adenocarcinomas. Tumors grossly form a firm indurated mass presenting a "barrel-shaped" cervix. Tumor cells have abundant clear or pale eosinophilic cytoplasm and distinct cell borders (Fig. 2.2c). Various degrees of cytological and architectural atypia are seen from minimal in MDA and to prominent in poorly differentiated type. Neoplastic glands haphazardly infiltrate deep into the cervical wall. LEGH and AIS of gastric type are frequently seen in association with the tumor. The tumor is positive for HIK1083 and MUC6, markers of gastric pyloric gland differentiation [45, 46] (Fig. 2.2d). Most cases are negative for p16. Some tumors are diffusely positive or completely negative for p53 [47]. ER and PgR expression is negative [48]. Differential diagnosis of MDA and LEGH is often challenging. Immunohistochemical features including HIK1083, MUC6, and p16 expression overlap between the two lesions. LEGH is typically located in the superior portion of the cervix close to the internal os [49]. The lesion is usually confined to the superficial half of the cervical wall with characteristic lobular arrangement of small glands surrounding a large cyst [50, 51] (Fig. 2.3c). MDA arises in the transformation zone and extends widely throughout the cervix with a haphazard infiltrative pattern.

Intestinal type is characterized by the presence of goblet cells. Paneth cells and argentaffin cells may also be seen. Colloid carcinoma with prominent extracellular mucin is rarely observed [52]. Signet-ring cell type of the uterine cervix is extremely rare. The diagnosis should be made only after exclusion of metastatic carcinoma from the stomach, breast, and other digestive organs [53, 54].

Various types of benign pseudoneoplastic glandular lesions should be differentiated from mucinous carcinoma. Type A (non-cystic) tunnel clusters and diffuse laminar endocervical glandular hyperplasia show florid proliferation of endocervical glands. Both lesions lack significant cytological atypia and haphazard invasive growth. Type A tunnel cluster is usually seen in multigravida women and has characteristic lobulated arrangement of small glands [55]. Type A tunnel cluster may be positive for gastric-type mucin [56]. Diffuse laminar endocervical glandular hyperplasia is confined to the inner third of the cervical wall and shows evenly spaced proliferation of moderate-sized glands [57]. Microglandular hyperplasia is a common benign lesion characterized by closely packed proliferation of small glands [58] (Fig. 2.3d). The glands are lined by endocervical-like columnar cells with subnuclear or supranuclear vacuoles and contain neutrophils. Reserve cell hyperplasia and squamous metaplasia are usually admixed with glandular proliferation. Endocervical adenomyoma is a polypoid lesion characterized by florid proliferation of endocervical glands surrounded by smooth muscle (Fig. 2.3e). The glands are arranged in a lobular pattern and without cytological atypia [59]. Deep nabothian cysts, florid cystic endosalpingiosis, and endocervicosis are benign glands involving the deep cervical wall [60]. These lesions lack cytological atypia and infiltrative growth with stromal reaction.

2.3.3.3 Villoglandular Carcinoma

Villoglandular carcinoma is an architecturally defined subtype with an exophytic, villous/papillary growth pattern [61]. It is considered a rare variant of endocervical adenocarcinoma, usual type [12]. Patients with villoglandular carcinoma are relatively young with a mean age of 35 years. Neoplastic

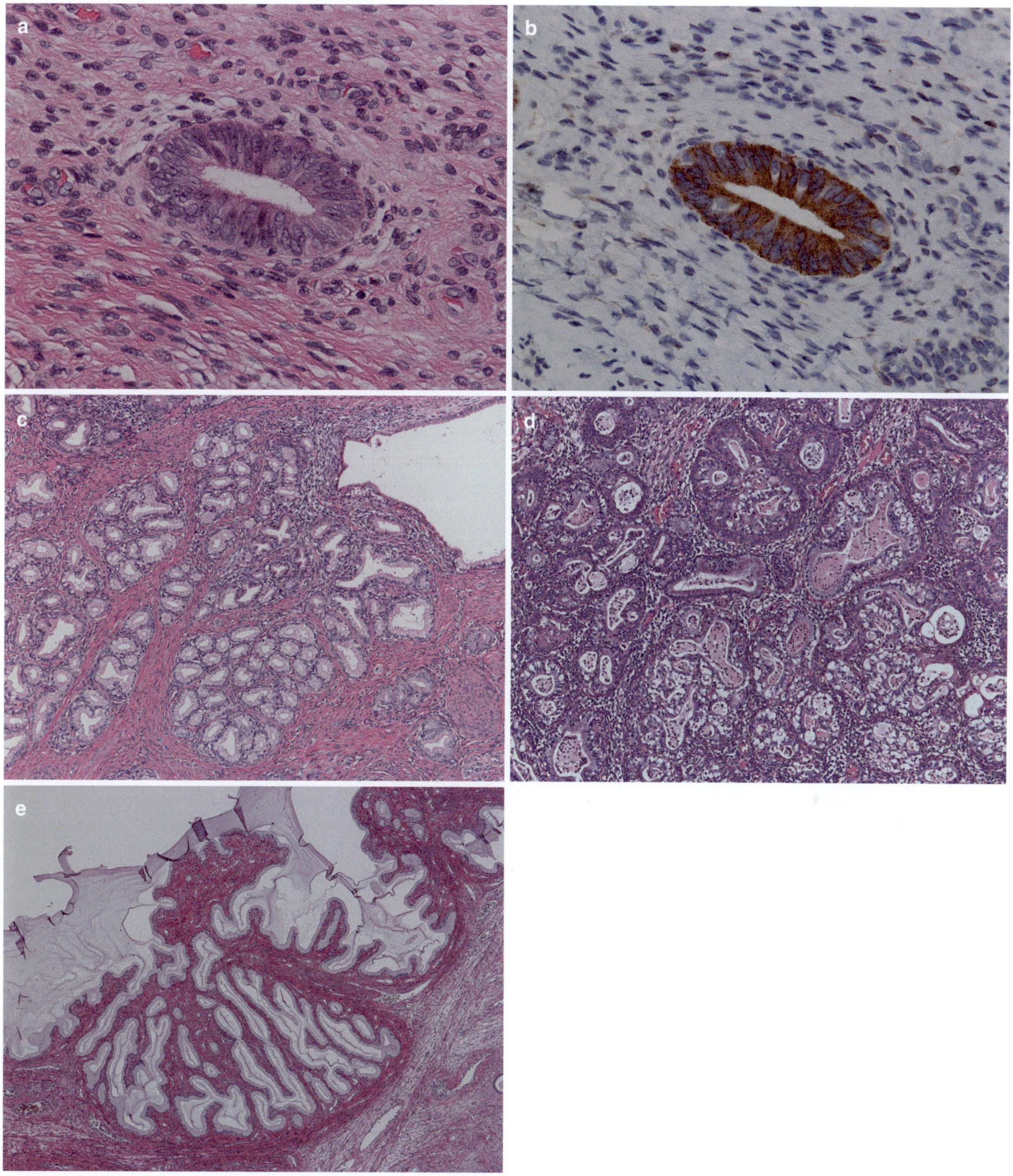

Fig. 2.3 Pseudoneoplastic glandular lesions. (**a**) Tuboendometrial metaplasia. (**b**) bcl-2 expression in tuboendometrial metaplasia. (**c**) Lobular endocervical glandular hyperplasia (LEGH). (**d**) Microglandular hyperplasia. (**e**) Endocervical adenomyoma

cells are tall and columnar-shaped with nuclear pseudostratification. Nuclear atypia is mild to moderate at most. At the surface, the tumor grows in a slender villous or papillary pattern with thin fibrovascular core (Fig. 2.2a). At the infiltrative portion, the tumor forms elongated tubular structures with complex intraluminal papillary growth and irregular branching. Villoglandular carcinoma is less aggressive than other types of cervical adenocarcinoma. Conservative surgery is an option for young patients who desire preservation of fertility if the tumor is confined to the surface, and the entire tumor consists of low-grade tumor cells [62, 63]. The diagnosis of villoglandular carcinoma should be restricted to a pure lesion with low-grade nuclei because other more aggressive types of cervical adenocarcinoma can exhibit focal villoglandular papillary architectures [41].

2.3.3.4 Endometrioid Carcinoma

Endometrioid carcinoma is defined as a cervical adenocarcinoma resembling endometrial endometrioid carcinoma. The tumor has well-formed tubular structures lined by columnar cells with prominent nuclear stratification and high N/C ratio. Intracytoplasmic mucin is absent (Fig. 2.2e). Cilia may be seen at the luminal surface. Nuclear grade and frequency of mitosis and apoptosis are less prominent compared with endocervical adenocarcinoma, usual type [64]. There are no universally accepted criteria to differentiate endometrioid carcinoma from endocervical adenocarcinoma, usual type. The ambiguity of diagnostic criteria is reflected by the wide range of incidence rates of cervical endometrioid carcinoma reported by various groups [65–68]. Endometrioid carcinoma of the cervix is currently considered to be rare with an incidence of no more than 5% [3]. Rare endometrioid carcinoma arises from cervical endometriosis. Cervical endometrioid carcinoma should be differentiated from cervical extension of endometrial endometrioid carcinoma. Endometrial endometrioid carcinoma is positive for ER and PgR, whereas cervical endometrioid carcinoma is typically negative for these markers. Vimentin is also more frequently positive in endometrial than cervical endometrioid carcinoma [11, 29]. p16 expression is diffuse and strongly positive in cervical endometrioid carcinoma but exhibits a patchy and heterogenous pattern in endometrial endometrioid carcinoma [69].

2.3.3.5 Clear Cell Carcinoma

Clear cell carcinoma is known for its association with diethylstilbestrol (DES) and occurrence in younger individuals (mean age, 19 years). Tumors in this setting characteristically arise in the exocervix and have a better prognosis [70]. After removal of DES from the market, cases of clear cell carcinoma have mainly occurred in older individuals similar to endocervical adenocarcinoma, usual type. DES-unrelated clear cell carcinoma shares similar clinical features with endocervical adenocarcinoma, usual type. Association with high-risk HPV is less frequent than endocervical adenocarcinoma, usual type [39, 40, 71]. Similar to its ovarian counterpart, the tumor grows in a tubulocystic, papillary, and solid pattern (Fig. 2.2f). Tumor cells are cuboidal, flat, and polygonal with clear or eosinophilic cytoplasm. Tubulocystic spaces may be lined by hobnail cells. The tumor also contains papillary structures with a hyalinized stromal core. Arias-Stella reaction should be differentiated from clear cell carcinoma. The clinical presentation of pregnancy or similar hormonal status is the most important clue. Arias-Stella reaction lacks solid and papillary growth and has a spectrum of cytologic atypia from bland to highly atypical [60].

2.3.3.6 Serous Carcinoma

Primary serous carcinoma of the cervix is very rare and should be diagnosed only after metastasis and/or direct extension from the ovary, and other female genital organs are excluded. The clinicopathological features are not significantly different from those of other types of cervical adenocarcinoma [72]. The histological findings are similar to ovarian or uterine counterparts. Serous carcinoma may be mixed with other types of cervical adenocarcinoma.

2.3.3.7 Mesonephric Carcinoma

Mesonephric carcinoma arises in the mesonephric remnant which is located in the deep lateral cervical wall. There is no association with high-risk HPV infection [40, 73]. Mesonephric carcinoma has a wide age of onset, with a mean age of approximately 50 years [74–76]. Abnormal uterine bleeding is the common clinical presentation. Grossly the tumor is an intramural large mass that frequently involves the lower uterine segment. Histologically, various growth patterns are seen including tubular, ductal, retiform, solid, and sex cord-like patterns. Tubular patterns are characterized by a proliferation of small round tubules lined by cuboidal or flat epithelial cells containing deep eosinophilic secretion (Fig. 2.2g). Ductal patterns resemble endometrioid carcinoma composed of tall columnar cells. Focal sarcomatous component may be observed [74, 76]. Mesonephric hyperplasia is frequently seen in the background. Although mesonephric carcinoma is not associated with HPV, p16 is positive in some cases. ER, PgR, and CEA are usually negative. More than 90% of mesonephric carcinomas are positive for GATA-binding protein 3 (GATA3), whereas most other cervical adenocarcinomas are negative. Some cases are positive for CD10, calretinin, and vimentin [76, 77]. Mesonephric hyperplasia is one of the more challenging diagnoses [78]. It is usually asymptomatic and the lesion is not grossly remarkable. Cytological atypia, irregularity of architecture, and glandular crowding are more prominent in carcinoma than in hyperplasia.

2.3.3.8 Adenocarcinoma Admixed with Neuroendocrine Carcinoma

Neuroendocrine carcinomas can be admixed with various types of cervical adenocarcinoma [79–81]. Small cell carcinoma and large cell neuroendocrine carcinomas are common, whereas carcinoid tumors are rare. The histological findings of neuroendocrine carcinomas are the same as those of lung counterpart. It should be noted that a minority of cervical neuroendocrine carcinomas are positive for TTF-1 [82]. Some cases are associated with high-risk HPV and p16 expression [80]; thus a common origin for adenocarcinoma and neuroendocrine carcinoma has been suggested [79].

References

1. Pirog EC, Lloveras B, Molijn A, Tous S, Guimera N, Alejo M, et al. HPV prevalence and genotypes in different histological subtypes of cervical adenocarcinoma, a worldwide analysis of 760 cases. Mod Pathol. 2014;27(12):1559–67.
2. Quint KD, de Koning MN, van Doorn LJ, Quint WG, Pirog EC. HPV genotyping and HPV16 variant analysis in glandular and squamous neoplastic lesions of the uterine cervix. Gynecol Oncol. 2010;117(2):297–301.
3. Kurman RJ, Carcangiu ML, Herrington CS, Young RH. WHO classification of tumours of female reproductive organs. 4th ed. International Agency for Research on Cancer; 2014. 307 p.
4. Friedell GH, McKay KD. Adenocarcinoma in situ of the endocervix. Cancer. 1953;6(5):887–97.
5. Gloor E, Hurlimann J. Cervical intraepithelial glandular neoplasia (adenocarcinoma in situ and glandular dysplasia). A correlative study of 23 cases with histologic grading, histochemical analysis of mucins, and immunohistochemical determination of the affinity for four lectins. Cancer. 1986;58(6):1272–80.
6. Ostor AG, Duncan A, Quinn M, Rome R. Adenocarcinoma in situ of the uterine cervix: an experience with 100 cases. Gynecol Oncol. 2000;79(2):207–10.
7. Tavassoli FA, Devilee P, International Agency for Research on Cancer, World Health Organization. Pathology and genetics of tumours of the breast and female genital organs. International Agency for Research on Cancer; 2003. 432 p.
8. Ioffe OB, Sagae S, Moritani S, Dahmoush L, Chen TT, Silverberg SG. Proposal of a new scoring scheme for the diagnosis of noninvasive endocervical glandular lesions. Am J Surg Pathol. 2003;27(4):452–60.
9. Goldstein NS, Ahmad E, Hussain M, Hankin RC, Perez-Reyes N. Endocervical glandular atypia: does a preneoplastic lesion of adenocarcinoma in situ exist? Am J Clin Pathol. 1998;110(2):200–9.
10. Lee KR. Symposium part 4: should pathologists diagnose endocervical preneoplastic lesions "less than" adenocarcinoma in situ?: Counterpoint. Int J Gynecol Pathol. 2003;22(1):22–4.
11. Zaino RJ. Glandular lesions of the uterine cervix. Mod Pathol. 2000;13(3):261–74.
12. Loureiro J, Oliva E. The spectrum of cervical glandular neoplasia and issues in differential diagnosis. Arch Pathol Lab Med. 2014;138(4):453–83.
13. Witkiewicz A, Lee KR, Brodsky G, Cviko A, Brodsky J, Crum CP. Superficial (early) endocervical adenocarcinoma in situ: a study of 12 cases and comparison to conventional AIS. Am J Surg Pathol. 2005;29(12):1609–14.
14. Bertrand M, Lickrish GM, Colgan TJ. The anatomic distribution of cervical adenocarcinoma in situ: implications for treatment. Am J Obstet Gynecol. 1987;157(1):21–5.
15. Jaworski RC, Pacey NF, Greenberg ML, Osborn RA. The histologic diagnosis of adenocarcinoma in situ and related lesions of the cervix uteri. Adenocarcinoma in situ. Cancer. 1988;61(6):1171–81.
16. Jaworski RC. Endocervical glandular dysplasia, adenocarcinoma in situ, and early invasive (microinvasive) adenocarcinoma of the uterine cervix. Semin Diagn Pathol. 1990;7(3):190–204.
17. Moritani S, Ioffe OB, Sagae S, Dahmoush L, Silverberg SG, Hattori T. Mitotic activity and apoptosis in endocervical glandular lesions. Int J Gynecol Pathol. 2002;21(2):125–33.
18. Park JJ, Sun D, Quade BJ, Flynn C, Sheets EE, Yang A, et al. Stratified mucin-producing intraepithelial lesions of the cervix: adenosquamous or columnar cell neoplasia? Am J Surg Pathol. 2000;24(10):1414–9.
19. Schlesinger C, Silverberg SG. Endocervical adenocarcinoma in situ of tubal type and its relation to atypical tubal metaplasia. Int J Gynecol Pathol. 1999;18(1):1–4.
20. Mikami Y, McCluggage WG. Endocervical glandular lesions exhibiting gastric differentiation: an emerging spectrum of benign, premalignant, and malignant lesions. Adv Anat Pathol. 2013;20(4):227–37.
21. Kong CS, Beck AH, Longacre TA. A panel of 3 markers including p16, ProExC, or HPV ISH is optimal for distinguishing between primary endometrial and endocervical adenocarcinomas. Am J Surg Pathol. 2010;34(7):915–26.
22. Negri G, Bellisano G, Carico E, Faa G, Kasal A, Antoniazzi S, et al. Usefulness of p16ink4a, ProEX C, and Ki-67 for the diagnosis of glandular dysplasia and adenocarcinoma of the cervix uteri. Int J Gynecol Pathol. 2011;30(4):407–13.
23. McCluggage G, McBride H, Maxwell P, Bharucha H. Immunohistochemical detection of p53 and bcl-2 proteins in neoplastic and non-neoplastic endocervical glandular lesions. Int J Gynecol Pathol. 1997;16(1):22–7.
24. Baker PM, Clement PB, Bell DA, Young RH. Superficial endometriosis of the uterine cervix: a report of 20 cases of a process that may be confused with endocervical glandular dysplasia or adenocarcinoma in situ. Int J Gynecol Pathol. 1999;18(3):198–205.
25. Phadnis SV, Doshi JS, Ogunnaike O, Coady A, Padwick M, Sanusi FA. Cervical endometriosis: a diagnostic and management dilemma. Arch Gynecol Obstet. 2005;272(4):289–93.
26. Jonasson JG, Wang HH, Antonioli DA, Ducatman BS. Tubal metaplasia of the uterine cervix: a prevalence study in patients with gynecologic pathologic findings. Int J Gynecol Pathol. 1992;11(2):89–95.
27. Cameron RI, Maxwell P, Jenkins D, McCluggage WG. Immunohistochemical staining with MIB1, bcl2 and p16 assists in the distinction of cervical glandular intraepithelial neoplasia from tubo-endometrial metaplasia, endometriosis and microglandular hyperplasia. Histopathology. 2002;41(4):313–21.
28. McCluggage WG, Maxwell P. Bcl-2 and p21 immunostaining of cervical tubo-endometrial metaplasia. Histopathology. 2002;40(1):107–8.
29. Staebler A, Sherman ME, Zaino RJ, Ronnett BM. Hormone receptor immunohistochemistry and human papillomavirus in situ hybridization are useful for distinguishing endocervical and endometrial adenocarcinomas. Am J Surg Pathol. 2002;26(8):998–1006.
30. McCluggage WG, Jenkins D. p16 immunoreactivity may assist in the distinction between endometrial and endocervical adenocarcinoma. Int J Gynecol Pathol. 2003;22(3):231–5.
31. O'Neill CJ, McCluggage WG. p16 expression in the female genital tract and its value in diagnosis. Adv Anat Pathol. 2006;13(1):8–15.
32. Schorge JO, Lee KR, Flynn CE, Goodman A, Sheets EE. Stage IA1 cervical adenocarcinoma: definition and treatment. Obstet Gynecol. 1999;93(2):219–22.
33. Matsukuma K, Tsukamoto N, Kaku T, Matsumura M, Toki N, Toh N, et al. Early adenocarcinoma of the uterine cervix—its histologic and immunohistologic study. Gynecol Oncol. 1989;35(1):38–43.
34. Ostor A, Rome R, Quinn M. Microinvasive adenocarcinoma of the cervix: a clinicopathologic study of 77 women. Obstet Gynecol. 1997;89(1):88–93.
35. Mulvany N, Ostor A. Microinvasive adenocarcinoma of the cervix: a cytohistopathologic study of 40 cases. Diagn Cytopathol. 1997;16(5):430–6.
36. Teshima S, Shimosato Y, Kishi K, Kasamatsu T, Ohmi K, Uei Y. Early stage adenocarcinoma of the uterine cervix. Histopathologic analysis with consideration of histogenesis. Cancer. 1985;56(1):167–72.
37. Kaspar HG, Dinh TV, Doherty MG, Hannigan EV, Kumar D. Clinical implications of tumor volume measurement in stage I adenocarcinoma of the cervix. Obstet Gynecol. 1993;81(2):296–300.
38. Karamurzin YS, Kiyokawa T, Parkash V, Jotwani AR, Patel P, Pike MC, et al. Gastric-type endocervical adenocarcinoma: an aggressive tumor with unusual metastatic patterns and poor prognosis. Am J Surg Pathol. 2015;39(11):1449–57.

39. Pirog EC, Kleter B, Olgac S, Bobkiewicz P, Lindeman J, Quint WG, et al. Prevalence of human papillomavirus DNA in different histological subtypes of cervical adenocarcinoma. Am J Pathol. 2000;157(4):1055–62.
40. Park KJ, Kiyokawa T, Soslow RA, Lamb CA, Oliva E, Zivanovic O, et al. Unusual endocervical adenocarcinomas: an immunohistochemical analysis with molecular detection of human papillomavirus. Am J Surg Pathol. 2011;35(5):633–46.
41. Young RH, Clement PB. Endocervical adenocarcinoma and its variants: their morphology and differential diagnosis. Histopathology. 2002;41(3):185–207.
42. Kojima A, Mikami Y, Sudo T, Yamaguchi S, Kusanagi Y, Ito M, et al. Gastric morphology and immunophenotype predict poor outcome in mucinous adenocarcinoma of the uterine cervix. Am J Surg Pathol. 2007;31(5):664–72.
43. Kusanagi Y, Kojima A, Mikami Y, Kiyokawa T, Sudo T, Yamaguchi S, et al. Absence of high-risk human papillomavirus (HPV) detection in endocervical adenocarcinoma with gastric morphology and phenotype. Am J Pathol. 2010;177(5):2169–75.
44. Kawauchi S, Kusuda T, Liu XP, Suehiro Y, Kaku T, Mikami Y, et al. Is lobular endocervical glandular hyperplasia a cancerous precursor of minimal deviation adenocarcinoma?: a comparative molecular-genetic and immunohistochemical study. Am J Surg Pathol. 2008;32(12):1807–15.
45. Mikami Y, Kiyokawa T, Hata S, Fujiwara K, Moriya T, Sasano H, et al. Gastrointestinal immunophenotype in adenocarcinomas of the uterine cervix and related glandular lesions: a possible link between lobular endocervical glandular hyperplasia/pyloric gland metaplasia and 'adenoma malignum'. Mod Pathol. 2004;17(8):962–72.
46. Ishii K, Hosaka N, Toki T, Momose M, Hidaka E, Tsuchiya S, et al. A new view of the so-called adenoma malignum of the uterine cervix. Virchows Arch. 1998;432(4):315–22.
47. Carleton C, Hoang L, Sah S, Kiyokawa T, Karamurzin YS, Talia KL, et al. A detailed Immunohistochemical analysis of a large series of cervical and vaginal gastric-type adenocarcinomas. Am J Surg Pathol. 2016;40(5):636–44.
48. McCluggage WG. Recent developments in non-HPV-related adenocarcinomas of the lower female genital tract and their precursors. Adv Anat Pathol. 2016;23(1):58–69.
49. Sasajima Y, Mikami Y, Kaku T, Kiyokawa T, Ohishi Y, Hamada T, et al. Gross features of lobular endocervical glandular hyperplasia in comparison with minimal-deviation adenocarcinoma and stage Ib endocervical-type mucinous adenocarcinoma of the uterine cervix. Histopathology. 2008;53(4):487–90.
50. Nucci MR. Pseudoneoplastic glandular lesions of the uterine cervix: a selective review. Int J Gynecol Pathol. 2014;33(4):330–8.
51. Nucci MR, Clement PB, Young RH. Lobular endocervical glandular hyperplasia, not otherwise specified: a clinicopathologic analysis of thirteen cases of a distinctive pseudoneoplastic lesion and comparison with fourteen cases of adenoma malignum. Am J Surg Pathol. 1999;23(8):886–91.
52. Shintaku M, Kushima R, Abiko K. Colloid carcinoma of the intestinal type in the uterine cervix: mucin immunohistochemistry. Pathol Int. 2010;60(2):119–24.
53. Cracchiolo B, Kuhn T, Heller D. Primary signet ring cell adenocarcinoma of the uterine cervix—a rare neoplasm that raises the question of metastasis to the cervix. Gynecol Oncol Rep. 2016;16:9–10.
54. Imachi M, Tsukamoto N, Amagase H, Shigematsu T, Amada S, Nakano H. Metastatic adenocarcinoma to the uterine cervix from gastric cancer. A clinicopathologic analysis of 16 cases. Cancer. 1993;71(11):3472–7.
55. Fluhmann CF. Focal hyperplasis (tunnel clusters) of the cervix uteri. Obstet Gynecol. 1961;17:206–14.
56. Kondo T, Hashi A, Murata SI, Fischer SE, Nara M, Nakazawa T, et al. Gastric mucin is expressed in a subset of endocervical tunnel clusters: type a tunnel clusters of gastric phenotype. Histopathology. 2007;50(7):843–50.
57. Jones MA, Young RH, Scully RE. Diffuse laminar endocervical glandular hyperplasia. A benign lesion often confused with adenoma malignum (minimal deviation adenocarcinoma). Am J Surg Pathol. 1991;15(12):1123–9.
58. Taylor HB, Irey NS, Norris HJ. Atypical endocervical hyperplasia in women taking oral contraceptives. JAMA. 1967;202(7):637–9.
59. Gilks CB, Young RH, Clement PB, Hart WR, Scully RE. A new view of the so-called adenoma malignum of the uterine cervix. Mod Pathol. 1996;9(3):220–4.
60. Nucci MR. Symposium part III: tumor-like glandular lesions of the uterine cervix. Int J Gynecol Pathol. 2002;21(4):347–59.
61. Young RH, Scully RE. Villoglandular papillary adenocarcinoma of the uterine cervix. A clinicopathologic analysis of 13 cases. Cancer. 1989;63(9):1773–9.
62. Jones MW, Silverberg SG, Kurman RJ. Well-differentiated villoglandular adenocarcinoma of the uterine cervix: a clinicopathological study of 24 cases. Int J Gynecol Pathol. 1993;12(1):1–7.
63. Falcon O, Garcia R, Lubrano A, Morin JC, Andujar M. Successful term delivery following conservative management for villoglandular papillary adenocarcinoma of the uterine cervix: a case report. Gynecol Oncol. 2006;101(1):168–71.
64. Clement PB, Young RH. Atlas of gynecologic surgical pathology. 3rd ed. Elsevier/Saunders; 2014. xi, 568 p.
65. Schorge JO, Lee KR, Lee SJ, Flynn CE, Goodman A, Sheets EE. Early cervical adenocarcinoma: selection criteria for radical surgery. Obstet Gynecol. 1999;94(3):386–90.
66. Alfsen GC, Thoresen SO, Kristensen GB, Skovlund E, Abeler VM. Histopathologic subtyping of cervical adenocarcinoma reveals increasing incidence rates of endometrioid tumors in all age groups: a population based study with review of all nonsquamous cervical carcinomas in Norway from 1966 to 1970, 1976 to 1980, and 1986 to 1990. Cancer. 2000;89(6):1291–9.
67. Wang SS, Sherman ME, Silverberg SG, Carreon JD, Lacey JV Jr, Zaino R, et al. Pathological characteristics of cervical adenocarcinoma in a multi-center US-based study. Gynecol Oncol. 2006;103(2):541–6.
68. Zaino RJ. The fruits of our labors: distinguishing endometrial from endocervical adenocarcinoma. Int J Gynecol Pathol. 2002;21(1):1–3.
69. Ansari-Lari MA, Staebler A, Zaino RJ, Shah KV, Ronnett BM. Distinction of endocervical and endometrial adenocarcinomas: immunohistochemical p16 expression correlated with human papillomavirus (HPV) DNA detection. Am J Surg Pathol. 2004;28(2):160–7.
70. Herbst AL. Behavior of estrogen-associated female genital tract cancer and its relation to neoplasia following intrauterine exposure to diethylstilbestrol (DES). Gynecol Oncol. 2000;76(2):147–56.
71. Kocken M, Baalbergen A, Snijders PJ, Bulten J, Quint WG, Smedts F, et al. High-risk human papillomavirus seems not involved in DES-related and of limited importance in nonDES related clear-cell carcinoma of the cervix. Gynecol Oncol. 2011;122(2):297–302.
72. Zhou C, Gilks CB, Hayes M, Clement PB. Papillary serous carcinoma of the uterine cervix: a clinicopathologic study of 17 cases. Am J Surg Pathol. 1998;22(1):113–20.
73. Kenny SL, McBride HA, Jamison J, McCluggage WG. Mesonephric adenocarcinomas of the uterine cervix and corpus: HPV-negative neoplasms that are commonly PAX8, CA125, and HMGA2 positive and that may be immunoreactive with TTF1 and hepatocyte nuclear factor 1-beta. Am J Surg Pathol. 2012;36(6):799–807.
74. Bague S, Rodriguez IM, Prat J. Malignant mesonephric tumors of the female genital tract: a clinicopathologic study of 9 cases. Am J Surg Pathol. 2004;28(5):601–7.
75. Ferry JA, Scully RE. Mesonephric remnants, hyperplasia, and neoplasia in the uterine cervix. A study of 49 cases. Am J Surg Pathol. 1990;14(12):1100–11.
76. Silver SA, Devouassoux-Shisheboran M, Mezzetti TP, Tavassoli FA. Mesonephric adenocarcinomas of the uterine cervix: a study

of 11 cases with immunohistochemical findings. Am J Surg Pathol. 2001;25(3):379–87.
77. McCluggage WG, Oliva E, Herrington CS, McBride H, Young RH. CD10 and calretinin staining of endocervical glandular lesions, endocervical stroma and endometrioid adenocarcinomas of the uterine corpus: CD10 positivity is characteristic of, but not specific for, mesonephric lesions and is not specific for endometrial stroma. Histopathology. 2003;43(2):144–50.
78. Jones MA, Andrews J, Tarraza HM. Mesonephric remnant hyperplasia of the cervix: a clinicopathologic analysis of 14 cases. Gynecol Oncol. 1993;49(1):41–7.
79. Cui S, Lespinasse P, Cracchiolo B, Sama J, Kreitzer MS, Heller DS. Large cell neuroendocrine carcinoma of the cervix associated with adenocarcinoma in situ: evidence of a common origin. Int J Gynecol Pathol. 2001;20(3):311–2.
80. Ramalingam P, Malpica A, Deavers MT. Mixed endocervical adenocarcinoma and high-grade neuroendocrine carcinoma of the cervix with ovarian metastasis of the former component: a report of 2 cases. Int J Gynecol Pathol. 2012;31(5):490–6.
81. Rekhi B, Patil B, Deodhar KK, Maheshwari A, A Kerkar R, Gupta S, et al. Spectrum of neuroendocrine carcinomas of the uterine cervix, including histopathologic features, terminology, immunohistochemical profile, and clinical outcomes in a series of 50 cases from a single institution in India. Ann Diagn Pathol. 2013;17(1):1–9.
82. Carlson JW, Nucci MR, Brodsky J, Crum CP, Hirsch MS. Biomarker-assisted diagnosis of ovarian, cervical and pulmonary small cell carcinomas: the role of TTF-1, WT-1 and HPV analysis. Histopathology. 2007;51(3):305–12.

Heterogeneity of the Precursor Lesions of Endometrial Carcinoma, According to the Histologic Subtype

3

Hiroyuki Yanai

Abstract

Endometrial carcinoma is a constellation of different types of carcinomas, each exhibiting different morphology, genetic abnormalities, and clinical outcomes and developing via a different carcinogenesis process. Atypical endometrial hyperplasia/endometrioid intraepithelial neoplasia (AEH/EIN) is a precursor of endometrioid carcinoma. AEH/EIN is a noninvasive proliferation of atypical epithelium, which frequently harbors mutations in the *PTEN*, *KRAS*, *CTNNB1*, or *ARID1A* genes that are observed in endometrioid carcinoma. Microsatellite instability caused by epigenetic suppression of DNA mismatch repair protein MLH1 is also observed in AEH/EIN. These genetic abnormalities constitute early events of endometrioid carcinogenesis. As serous carcinoma without stromal invasion shows aggressive behavior, noninvasive serous neoplasia is designated as serous endometrial intraepithelial carcinoma (SEIC). Mutation of *TP53* is detected in most cases of serous carcinoma and SEIC. Mutation of *TP53* occurs in normal-appearing epithelium and is designated as p53 signature. Some clear cell carcinomas have associated intraepithelial lesions exhibiting less atypia than carcinoma. Although this lesion is a putative precursor lesion of clear cell carcinoma, further study is necessary.

Keywords

Endometrial hyperplasia · Endometrioid intraepithelial neoplasia · Serous intraepithelial carcinoma · p53 signature · Clear cell carcinoma

3.1 Introduction

Endometrial carcinoma is not a single disease entity. In the 4th edition of the WHO classification, endometrial carcinoma is classified into endometrioid, mucinous, serous, clear cell, and other types of carcinomas. Historically, endometrial carcinoma has been divided into type I and type II based on pathogenetic features [1]. Type I tumors occur in women with obesity, hyperlipidemia, and signs of hyperestrogenism, and the background endometrium is usually hyperplastic. Type I tumors present in peri- or postmenopausal women and are usually histologically low grade with favorable clinical outcomes. In contrast, type II tumors arise in women lacking the abovementioned metabolic and endocrinological features. Type II tumors occur in atrophic endometrium and often exhibit high-grade morphological features and an aggressive clinical course. Moreover, patients of type II carcinoma are usually older than type I endometrial cancer patients. Interestingly, morphological classification and molecular abnormalities are well correlated with this two-tier classification. The prototype of type I tumors is low-grade endometrioid carcinoma and that of type II tumors is serous carcinoma. Clear cell carcinoma shows characteristics intermediate between endometrioid and serous carcinoma. Each type of endometrial carcinoma exhibits different morphological features and different molecular mechanisms and develops from unique precursor lesions.

In this chapter, the biology and diagnosis of precursor lesions of different types of endometrial carcinoma are discussed.

H. Yanai
Department of Pathology, Okayama University Hospital, Okayama, Japan
e-mail: yanaih@md.okayama-u.ac.jp

T. Moriya (ed.), *Pathology of Female Cancers*, https://doi.org/10.1007/978-981-10-8606-9_3

3.2 Precursors of Endometrioid Carcinoma

3.2.1 Endometrial Hyperplasia and Atypical Endometrial Hyperplasia

Endometrial endometrioid carcinoma is defined as an invasive carcinoma of the endometrium with proliferation of tumor cells, which are morphologically similar to the endometrial epithelium in the proliferative phase.

Endometrial epithelial proliferative lesions without invasive growth had been divided into endometrial hyperplasia (EH) and atypical endometrial hyperplasia (AEH), according to the cellular atypia of the glandular epithelium. EH shows proliferation of endometrial glands without cellular atypia and can be further divided into simple and complex types based on glandular complexity and density. Simple EH exhibits proliferation of glands with round-shaped and simple structures (Fig. 3.1a). Some glands may show outpouching. The stroma between glands is wide in simple EH. In contrast, complex EH is characterized by dense proliferation of irregular-shaped glands with budding or branching (Fig. 3.2). The stroma is narrower than that of simple EH. In most cases, EH is reactive hyperplastic lesion to hyperestrogenism. Instead of morphological difference, the rate of progression to carcinoma is less than 5% in both simple and complex EH patients [2]. Intra- and interobserver diagnostic reproducibility of simple and complex hyperplasia is unsatisfactory [3]. Thus, simple and complex EH are recognized as lesions in the spectrum of single disease entity, and subclassification of simple and complex EH is abolished in the 4th edition of the WHO classification [4].

AEH is EH superimposed by epithelial cellular atypia and lacks stromal invasion. Similar to EH, AEH can also be divided into simple and complex types based on glandular structure and density. Simple AEH is quite rare and AEH usually shows confluent proliferation of irregular-shaped glands. Atypia of AEH is mainly recognized by nuclear findings, i.e., loss of polarity, irregular stratification, nucleomegaly, round shape nuclei, prominent nucleolus, hyperchromatism, and coarse chromatin. Because the degree of nuclear atypia in AEH is similar to or at times higher than endometrioid carcinoma, nuclear atypia is not a reliable finding in the differential diagnosis of AEH and carcinoma [5].

Although AEH is defined clearly by cellular atypia and the absence of stromal invasion, recognition of these findings is subjective at times, and the diagnosis of AEH shows the lowest interobserver reproducibility among endometrial proliferative lesions [3, 6]. The panel diagnosis of the Gynecologic Oncology Group AEH study concurred with the referring diagnosis of AEH in only 39.8%, and the panel diagnosis was "less than AEH" in 25.6% and "carcinoma" in 29.1% of patients [7].

3.2.2 Endometrioid Intraepithelial Neoplasia (EIN)

Cumulative biological data regarding endometrial proliferative lesions indicate that some lesions constitute clonal proliferation of endometrial epithelium and definite precancerous lesions of endometrioid carcinoma. This means that these lesions represent neoplasia rather than hyperplasia. Mutter proposed the new diagnostic term, "endometrial intraepithelial neoplasia"

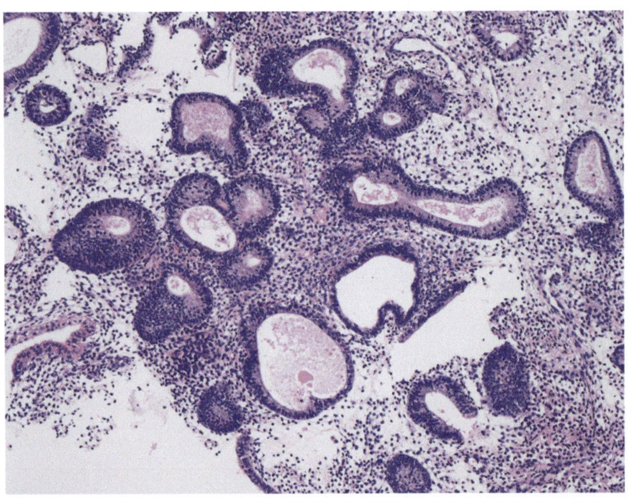

Fig. 3.1 Endometrial hyperplasia (simple). Glands are cystically dilated and mildly crowded. No significant atypia is noted. This pattern has been designated as simple hyperplasia

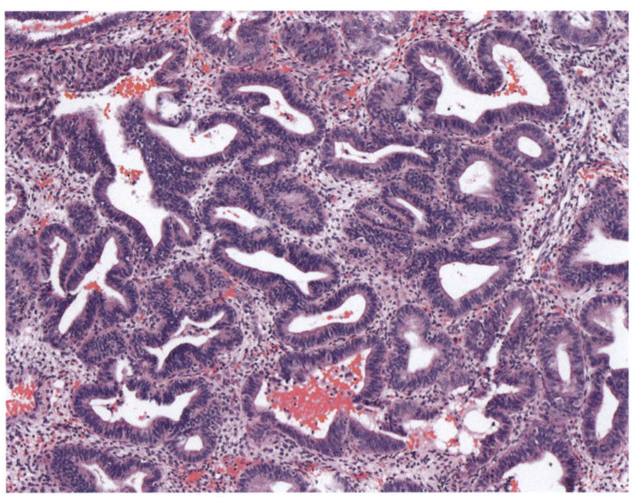

Fig. 3.2 Endometrial hyperplasia (complex). Complex hyperplasia shows dense proliferation of glands with complex shape. No significant atypia is noted

(EIN), which indicates true biological features [8]. Diagnostic criteria were established on the basis of morphological findings, genetic changes, morphometrical analysis, and clinical outcome. The EIN system scheme proposes that usage of the term "endometrial hyperplasia" should be limited to nonneoplastic proliferative lesions caused by unopposed or prolonged estrogen stimulus. The 4th edition of the WHO classification adopted the term "endometri*oid* intraepithelial neoplasia" instead of "endometri*al* intraepithelial neoplasia" [4]. This new term highlights that this lesion is a precursor of endometrioid carcinoma and not the other types of carcinoma.

An EIN diagnosis requires that the histological findings meet the following criteria (Table 3.1):

1. The area of the glands exceeds the area of stroma.
2. When a localizing lesion is present, epithelial cells within the architecturally crowded focus should be cytologically different compared to background glands.
3. The area meeting architectural and cytological criteria must have a minimum size of 1 mm.
4. Exclusion of both benign and malignant mimics (Figs. 3.3 and 3.4).

Table 3.1 Morphological diagnostic criteria of endometrial intraepithelial neoplasia (EIN)

Criterion	Findings
Architecture	Area of glands exceeds stroma
Cytology	Cytological findings of epithelium differ from background endometrial glands or apparently abnormal
Size	Maximum linear dimension is more than 1 mm
Exclude benign or malignant mimics	Basalis, secretory phase, polyp, etc.

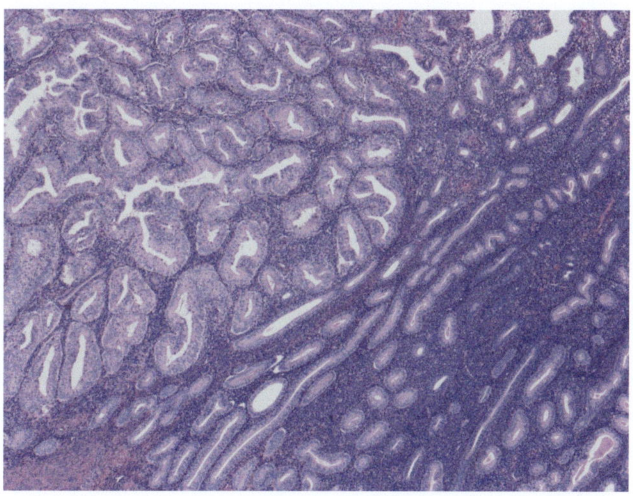

Fig. 3.3 Atypical endometrial hyperplasia/endometrioid intraepithelial neoplasia (AEH/EIN). Crowded proliferation of atypical glands (upper left) shows clear contrast to nonneoplastic region (lower right). In the lesion, area of glands exceeds stroma

The previous definitions of AEH (3rd edition of the WHO classification or former) and EIN proposed by Mutter are not interchangeable because of different diagnostic criteria. According to the study of Hecht et al., 78% of AEH are EIN and 64% of EIN are AEH; 29% and 7% of EIN cases correspond to complex and simple endometrial hyperplasia without atypia, respectively [9]. However, both terms appear as synonym in the 4th edition of the WHO classification [4].

3.2.3 Clinical Outcome of AEH and EIN

Several studies have addressed the clinical outcome of AEH. Rakha et al. reviewed these studies and found that 38% of biopsy- or curettage-identified AEHs are concurrent with endometrial carcinoma [10]. A study of their own series revealed that 27% of AEH cases had concurrent carcinoma; two thirds of these carcinomas were myoinvasive. In another study, 43% of AEH cases coexisted with carcinoma and 31% of these demonstrated myometrial invasion [7].

Baak et al. compared the rate of progression to carcinoma and found that an EIN diagnosis predicted progression more accurately than an AEH diagnosis [11].

3.2.4 Genetic Changes in AEH and EIN

Several different types of genetic abnormalities have been described in endometrioid carcinoma. Most endometrioid carcinomas have at least one mutation in the *PTEN*, *PIK3CA*, *KRAS*, *CTNNB1*, or *ARID1A* gene. Approximately 35% of endometrioid carcinomas display microsatellite instability (MSI). These genetic changes are also observed in the precursor lesions of endometrioid carcinoma.

Mutation of *PTEN* (phosphatase and tensin homolog deleted from chromosome 10), a tumor suppressor gene, is detected in 20–60% of AEH cases. *PTEN* encodes a phosphatase that catalyzes the dephosphorylation of phosphatidylinositol 3, 4, 5-trisphosphate. Mutation of *PTEN* causes the loss of function of this phosphatase, resulting in activation of the Akt pathway and accelerated cell proliferation. Sun et al. found a strong correlation between *PTEN* mutation and AEH clonality of AEH in combination and found strong correlation between them [12]. Hayes et al. showed that 48% of AEH cases harbored *PTEN* gene mutation [13]. Because mutation of *PTEN* causes the loss of PTEN protein expression in immunohistochemistry (IHC), PTEN IHC can serve as a substitute study and support the diagnosis of AEH/EIN. Loss of PTEN expression and gene mutations have been detected in 43% of normal-appearing endometrial glands, which could be latent precursors of EIN [14].

Mutation of *PIK3CA*, the gene encoding the catalytic p110-α subunit of phosphatidylinositol 3-kinase (PI3K), is

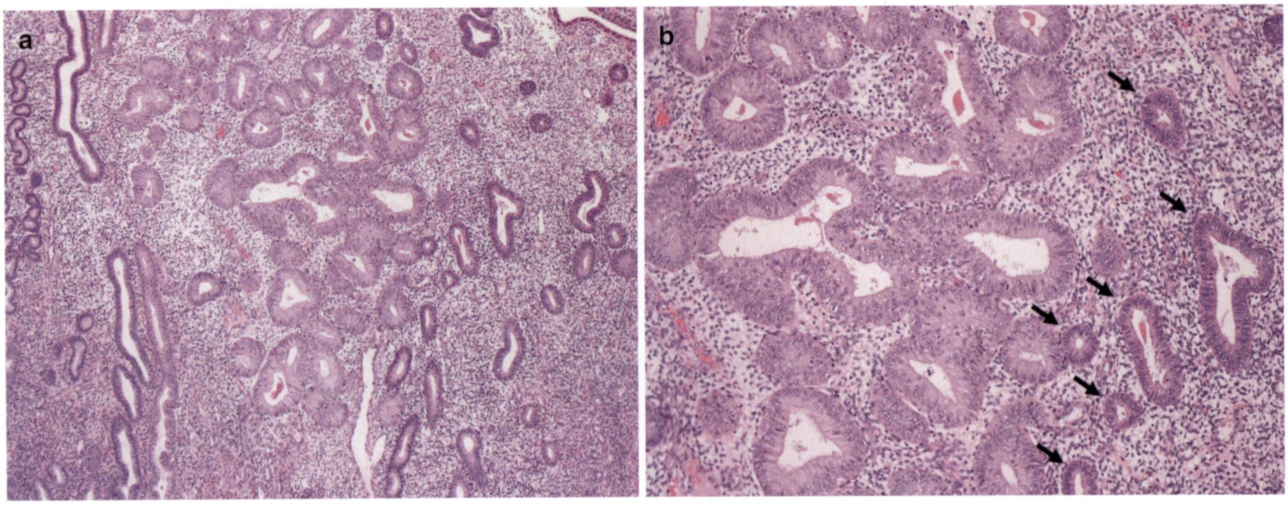

Fig. 3.4 Atypical endometrial hyperplasia/endometrioid intraepithelial neoplasia (AEH/EIN). (**a**) Size of lesion with crowded proliferation of atypical glands (middle) exceeds 1 mm, and size criteria of EIN are satisfied. (**b**) High-power view of (a) shows morphological difference between lesion and nonneoplastic glands (arrow)

frequently detected in endometrioid carcinoma. Majority of *PIK3CA* mutation occurs in exons 9 and 20 and results in activation of PI3K and Akt pathway. Mutation *PIK3CA* was detected in 7–22% of AEH cases [13, 15]. Konopka et al. reported that amplification of *PIK3CA* was found in 10% of AEH cases; however, they failed to detect mutations in this gene [16].

KRAS mutations have been detected in 16% of EIN cases [17]. Zauber et al. reported that 85.4% of AEHs accompanying *KRAS* mutated endometrioid carcinomas also harbor a *KRAS* mutation [18]. This finding indicates that *KRAS* mutations occur during an early step of endometrioid carcinogenesis.

Mutations in *CTNNB1*, the gene coding β-catenin, are common genetic abnormalities of endometrioid carcinoma. *CTNNB1* mutations are detected in 10–15% of AEH cases [19, 20]. This mutation causes nuclear localization of the β-catenin protein that can be recognized by IHC.

Mutation of *ARID1A* has been detected in some gynecological malignancies. *ARID1A* encodes the BAF250a protein, a component of the switch/sucrose non-fermenting (SWI/SNF) complex, which binds to DNA and participates in chromatin remodeling. Mutation of *ARID1A* results in loss of immunoreactivity; 20–40% cases of endometrial endometrioid carcinoma are negative for ARID1A immunostaining [21, 22]. Loss of ARID1A is detected in 16% of AEH cases but not in EH without atypia [22]. Mao et al. reported that the reduced expression of ARID1A is focal in AEH cases and there were no cases showing complete loss of AIRD1A [23]. These data indicate that mutation of *ARID1A* gene plays several roles in the early stage of endometrioid carcinogenesis and that it is a focal event in AEH.

DNA mismatch repair (MMR) abnormality is one of the major molecular mechanisms underlying endometrioid carcinoma. MMR deficiency is detected as MSI or the loss of MMR-related proteins (MLH1, PMS2, MSH2, MSH6, etc.) by IHC. MSI has been detected in about one third of endometrioid carcinoma and hyperplasia cases. The most frequent abnormality of MMR molecules is the loss of MLH1 protein expression caused by hypermethylation of the *MLH1* gene promoter region. MMR gene mutations also cause MSI and women with this mutation develop endometrial cancer (Lynch syndrome).

MMR deficiency has been detected in endometrial hyperplasia associated with endometrioid carcinoma, regardless of atypia. Cohn et al. reported that 83% of AEH cases associated with MSI-positive endometrial carcinoma were also MSI positive [24]. Han et al. showed the loss of at least one MMR molecule in more than half of complex endometrial hyperplasia cases [25]. Hypermethylation of the *MLH1* gene promoter has been detected in AEH [18]. These observations show that MSI caused by epigenetic suppression of MMR molecule expression is an early event of endometrioid carcinogenesis.

In contrast to serous carcinoma, mutation of *TP53* is not observed in most endometrioid carcinoma cases; although overexpression of p53 has been detected immunohistochemically, gene mutation of the *TP53* gene was not detected [26].

3.2.5 Differential Diagnosis of AEH and EIN

Both AEH and EIN should be differentiated from several benign lesions and carcinomas.

Benign conditions showing glandular crowding enter into differential diagnosis of AEH/EIN (Table 3.2). Because the basal layer of the normal endometrium exhibits crowding of glands and the morphological features of the epithelium differ from those of the functional layer, it should be differentiated from AEH/EIN (Fig. 3.5). During the mid-to-late secretory phase, the endometrium shows a reduced stromal area (Fig. 3.6). Menstruation history and associated stromal findings observed during the secretory phase, such as pseudodecidualization and spiral artery development, support the differential diagnosis. Some endometrial polyps contain areas with crowded glands; characteristic stromal features and careful evaluation of epithelial atypia support the diagnosis of endometrial polyps. Endometrial glandular and stromal breakdown (EGBD) exhibits gland crowding and associated epithelial metaplasia and results in a worrisome histological finding (Fig. 3.7). Stromal and epithelial apoptosis and fibrinous thrombi are characteristic findings of EGBD. Various types of epithelial metaplasia of the endometrium can be recognized as cellular atypia indicating EIN. The distinction between EH without atypia and AEH was discussed previously.

Atypical polypoid adenomyoma (APA) is a polypoid tumor composed of proliferation of atypical glands and

Table 3.2 Benign mimics of endometrial intraepithelial neoplasia

Conditions or lesions	Findings
Basalis	Crowded glands
Secretory phase	Crowded glands. In late secretory phase, stromal decidual change and spiral arteries are seen
Polyp	Focal glandular crowding or low proportion of stroma. Fibrous stroma
Endometrial glandular and stromal breakdown	Crowded glands. Epithelial metaplasia. Apoptosis in stroma and epithelium
Metaplasia	Difference of cellular appearance
Endometrial hyperplasia	Crowded glands. Lack cellular atypia
Atypical polypoid adenomyoma	Cellular atypia. Smooth muscle-like stroma

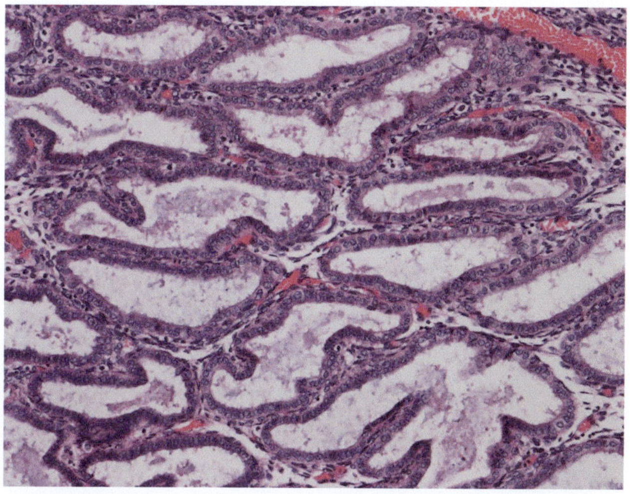

Fig. 3.6 Endometrium in secretory phase. An area of glands exceeds stroma (architecture criteria of EIN). Epithelial cells are cuboidal and cellular atypia is not seen

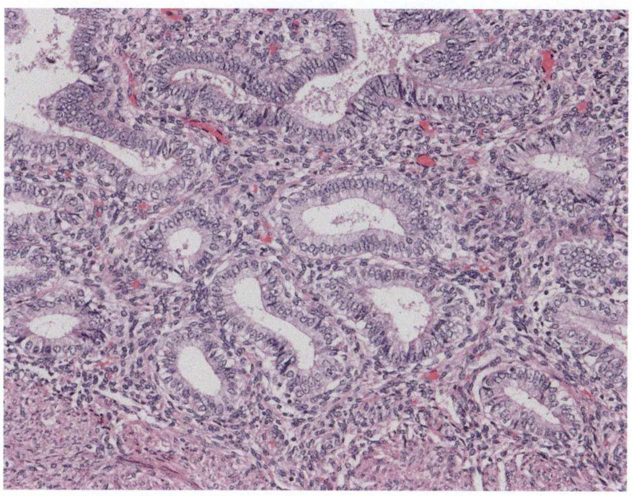

Fig. 3.5 Basalis of the endometrium. Glands are crowded. No cellular atypia is noted

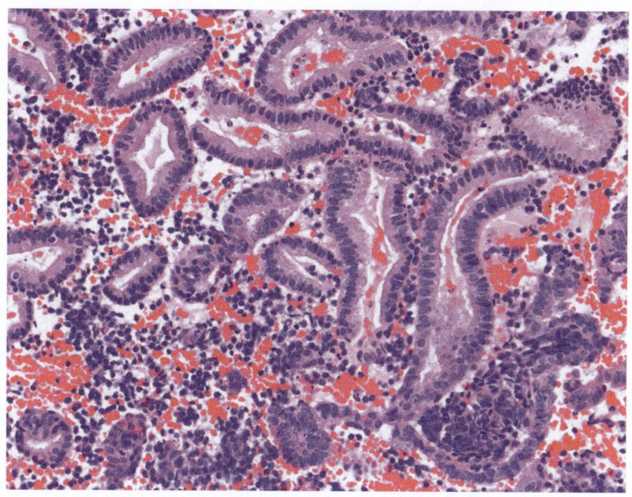

Fig. 3.7 Endometrial glandular and stromal breakdown. Although glands are crowded, stroma between glands is disorganized

smooth muscle-like stroma (Fig. 3.8). Stromal cells of APA have spindle and eosinophilic cytoplasm and resemble smooth muscle cells.

AEH/EIN should be distinguished from endometrioid carcinoma (Fig. 3.9). Since AEH lacks stromal invasion by definition, recognition of stromal invasion is key to the differential diagnosis between AEH/EIN and endometrioid carcinoma. Several criteria of stromal invasion have been proposed. Kurman and Norris have defined stromal invasion arbitrarily as follows: (1) an irregular infiltration of glands associated with an altered fibroblastic stroma or desmoplastic response; (2) a confluent glandular pattern in which individual glands, uninterrupted by stroma, merge and create a cribriform pattern; (3) an extensive papillary pattern; and (4) replacement of the stroma by masses of squamous epithelium [27]. In the 4th edition of WHO classification, stromal invasion is defined as the loss of intervening stroma (a confluent glandular or cribriform pattern) (Fig. 3.9a), an altered

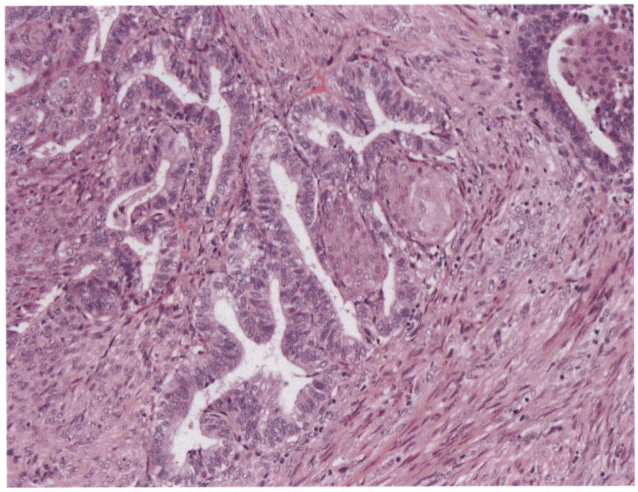

Fig. 3.8 Atypical polypoid adenomyoma. Proliferation of branching glands with morula formation is seen in the background of smooth muscle-like stroma

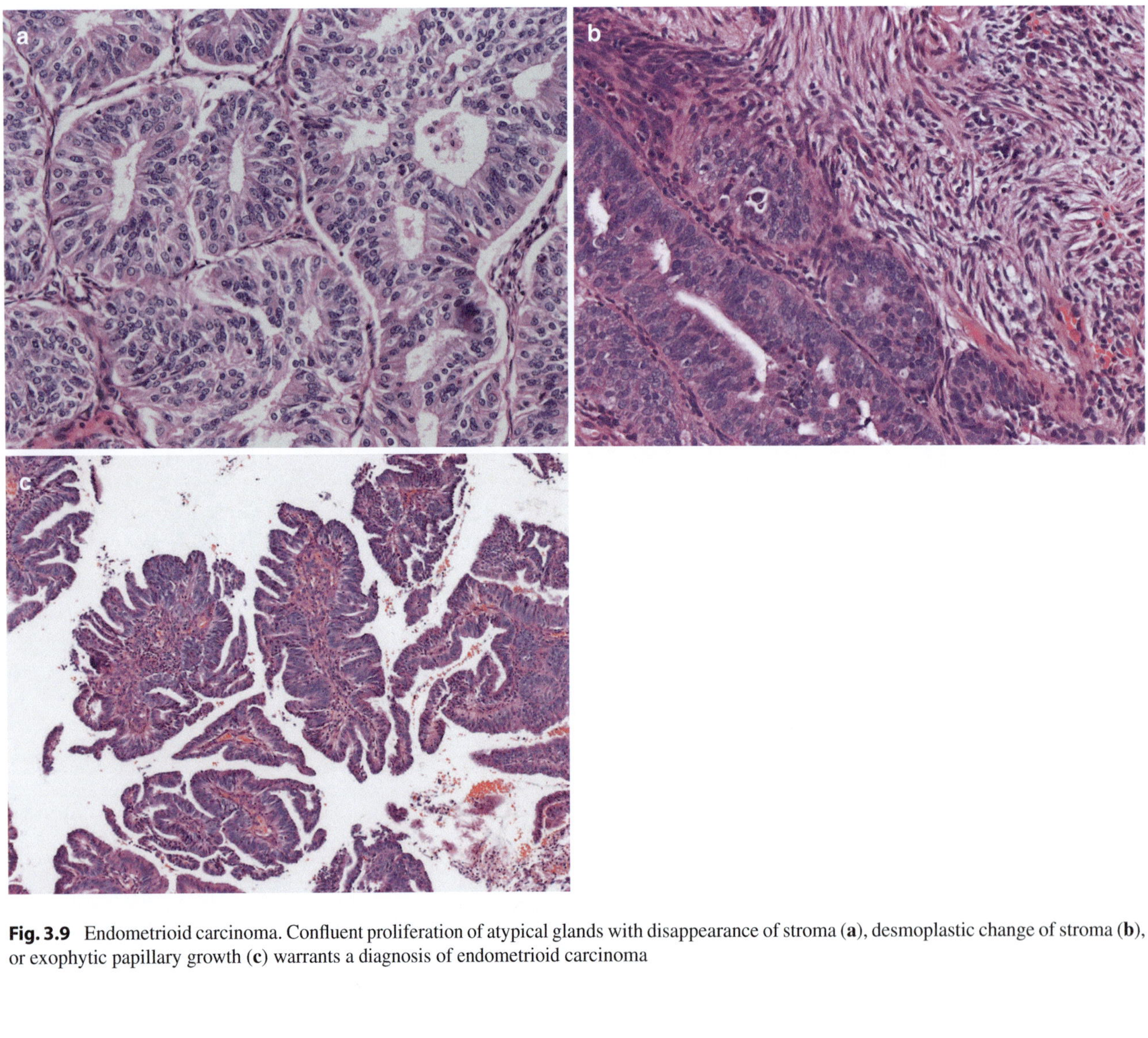

Fig. 3.9 Endometrioid carcinoma. Confluent proliferation of atypical glands with disappearance of stroma (**a**), desmoplastic change of stroma (**b**), or exophytic papillary growth (**c**) warrants a diagnosis of endometrioid carcinoma

endometrial stroma (desmoplastic reaction) (Fig. 3.9b), or a papillary architecture (villoglandular pattern) (Fig. 3.9c) [4]. Although myoinvasion is the most reliable finding of carcinoma, it is rarely found in curettage or biopsy specimens.

3.3 Precursors of Serous Carcinoma

Serous carcinoma of the endometrium is a prototype of type II endometrial carcinoma. It is defined as a carcinoma showing complex papillary and/or glandular architecture with diffuse, marked nuclear pleomorphism. The most characteristic molecular abnormality of serous carcinoma is mutation of *TP53*. Mutation of *TP53* causes aberrant p53 immunohistochemical status, abnormal accumulation of mutated p53 protein in nucleus, or complete lack of p53 immunoreactivity ("null" type). Abnormal p53 immunoreactivity suggests a diagnosis of serous carcinoma in morphologically problematic cases.

Serous carcinoma is often associated with noninvasive proliferation of carcinoma cells replacing surface or glandular epithelium. This condition has been designated as endometrial intraepithelial carcinoma [28]. Because serous carcinoma cells can spread to outside of the uterus through the fallopian tubes even in cases without stromal invasion and cause peritoneal carcinomatosis, serous tumor without stromal invasion warrants a carcinoma diagnosis [29].

3.3.1 Serous Endometrial Intraepithelial Carcinoma

Serous neoplasia without invasive growth is designated as serous endometrial intraepithelial carcinoma (SEIC). SEIC occurs in atrophic or weakly proliferative endometrium or endometrial polyp as multifocal lesions. SEIC is found in most uteri with serous carcinoma or carcinosarcoma with a serous epithelial component; however, it is only rarely observed in the background endometrium of endometrioid carcinoma or carcinosarcoma with an endometrioid epithelial component [28]. Because SEIC tumor cells proliferate and replace preexisting surface or glandular structure, the glandular density is not increased and stromal reactions such as desmoplasia are not evoked (Fig. 3.10). Cellular atypia of SEIC is similar to that of invasive serous carcinoma. The tumor cells are usually polygonal and sometimes hobnail-shaped and show marked nuclear atypia characterized by nucleomegaly, irregular shape, hyperchromatism, or prominent nucleolomegaly. Many mitotic figures are observed.

Similar to serous carcinoma, SEIC harbors mutation of *TP53* and p53 immunostain shows an aberrant pattern (Fig. 3.11) [30].

Expression of insulin-like growth factor II mRNA-binding protein 3 (IMP3) was observed in 94% of serous carcinoma and 89% of SEIC cases. These findings indicate that expression of IMP3 is an early event of serous carcinogenesis [31].

3.3.2 p53 Signature and Endometrial Glandular Dysplasia

The concept that precursor lesions of the ovarian high-grade serous carcinoma often arise in fimbria of the fallopian tube as serous tubal intraepithelial carcinoma (STIC) has gained wide acceptance recently. STICs exhibit marked cellular atypia and high proliferative capacity. STICs also exhibit aberrant p53 expression similar to ovarian high-grade serous carcinoma. A study examining p53 expression in the fallopian tubes has revealed that abnormal continuous p53 expression without cellular atypia or proliferative activity,

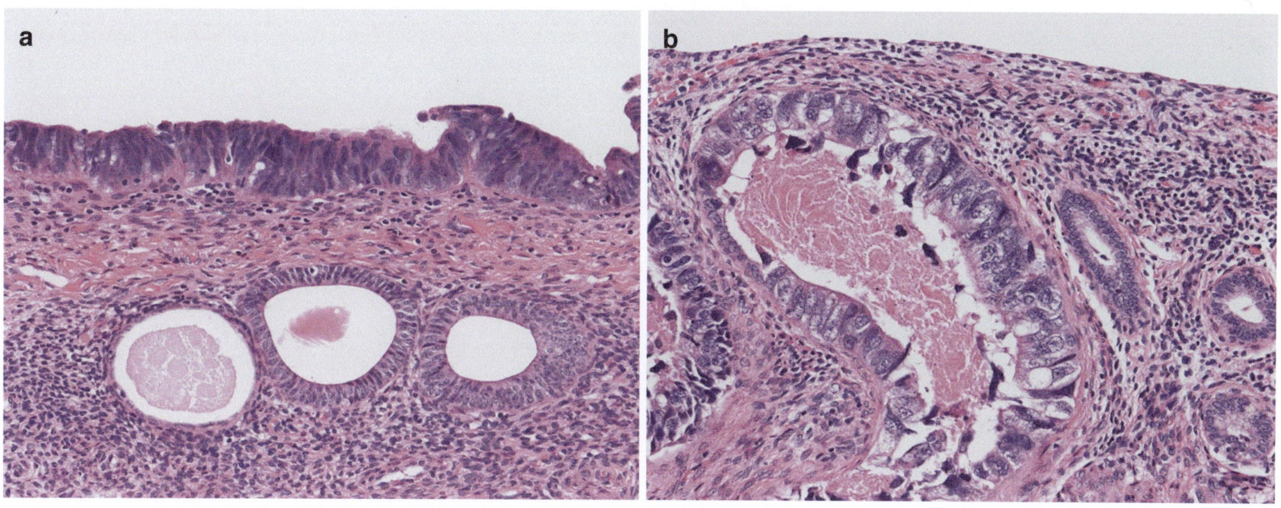

Fig. 3.10 Serous endometrial intraepithelial carcinoma. Highly atypical cells proliferate and replace surface (**a**) and/or glandular (**b**) epithelium

i.e., low Ki-67 index, is present in approximately one third of women without STIC; this status has been designated as the "p53 signature" [32].

An endometrial p53 signature has also been reported (Fig. 3.12) [33]; the p53 signature cannot be recognized morphologically and only IHC analysis of p53 can reveal this condition. The endometrial p53 signature was detected in 24% and 20% of the background endometrium of serous carcinoma and carcinosarcoma, respectively [34]. Similar to the tubal p53 signature, DNA damage, demonstrated by gamma-H2AX expression, was also found [33]. Moreover, *TP53* mutation was observed in 42% of endometrial p53 signature [35].

Some researchers have proposed the term "endometrial glandular dysplasia" (EmGD) to designate the lesion between the p53 signature and SEIC [36]. Morphologically, epithelial cells of glandular dysplasia show cellular atypia between resting endometrium and SEIC. The majority of EmGDs are multifocal and often found in uteri with serous carcinoma or SEIC but rarely found in uteri with endometrioid carcinoma. IHC of p53 and Ki-67 also demonstrates intermediate expression between resting endometrium and SEIC. IMP expression is observed in 14% of EmGDs [36]. Microdissected specimen of EmGDs revealed that 31.3% of the lesions show loss of heterogeneity at *TP53* locus [37]. These findings suggest that EmGD is a precursor of serous carcinoma; however, it falls short of serous EIC in terms of morphology and molecular biology. Establishment of diagnostic criteria with sufficient reproducibility will be the subject of future studies.

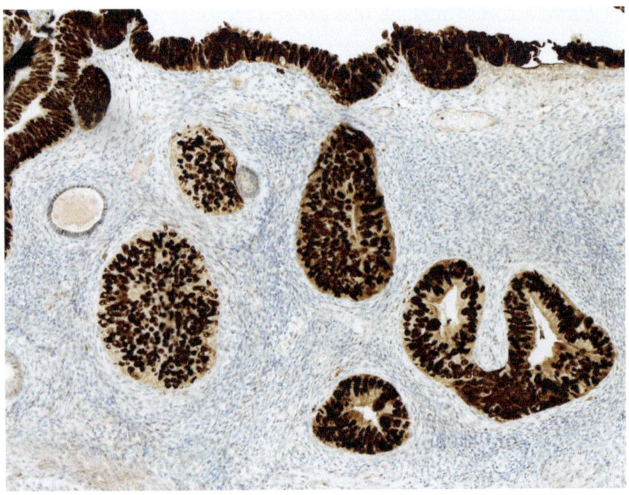

Fig. 3.11 Serous endometrial intraepithelial carcinoma. Carcinoma cells show aberrant expression of p53

3.4 Precursors of Clear Cell Carcinoma

Clear cell carcinoma is defined as a carcinoma showing characteristic papillary, solid, or tubulocystic proliferation of tumor cells with clear or eosinophilic cytoplasm or hobnail cells. The phenotype of clear cell carcinoma differs from that of endometrioid carcinoma or serous carcinoma. Clear cell carcinoma demonstrates immunonegativity for estrogen receptor (ER) and progesterone receptor (PgR), low p53 immunoreactivity, and high Ki-67 proliferative index [38]. Because clear cell carcinoma often coexists with endometrioid or serous carcinoma and identical gene mutations have been identified in both clear cell and non-clear cell components, endometrial clear cell carcinoma may develop via several tumorigenesis pathways.

Pure clear cell carcinoma is associated with AEH in 40% of cases, but not with SEIC [38]. Fadare et al. identified small glandular and/or surface intraepithelial lesions com-

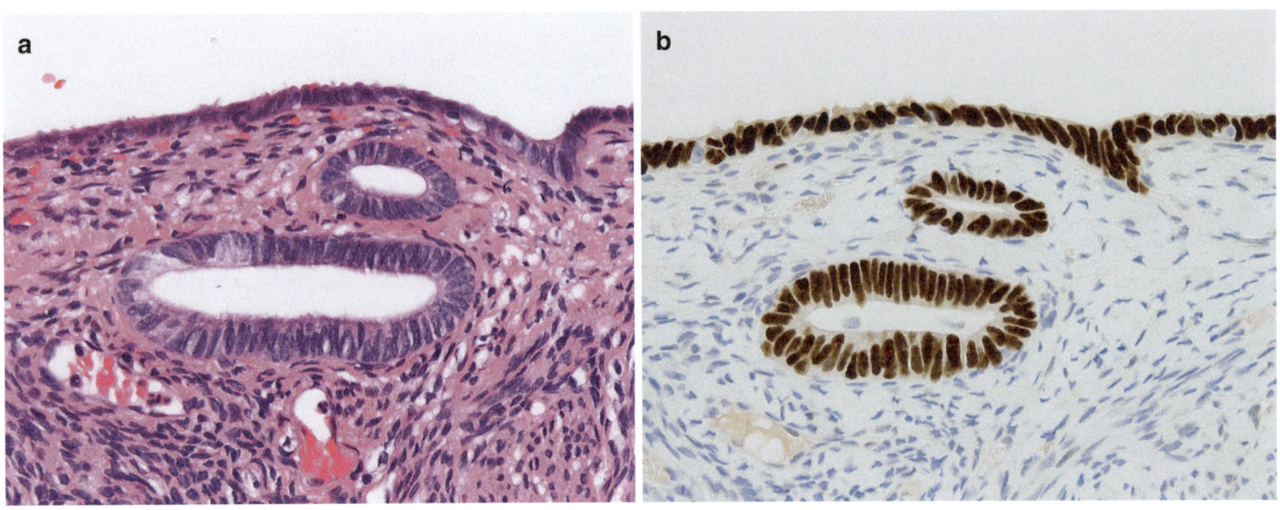

Fig. 3.12 p53 signature. Morphologically unremarkable glands (**a**) show strong and diffuse expression of p53 (**b**)

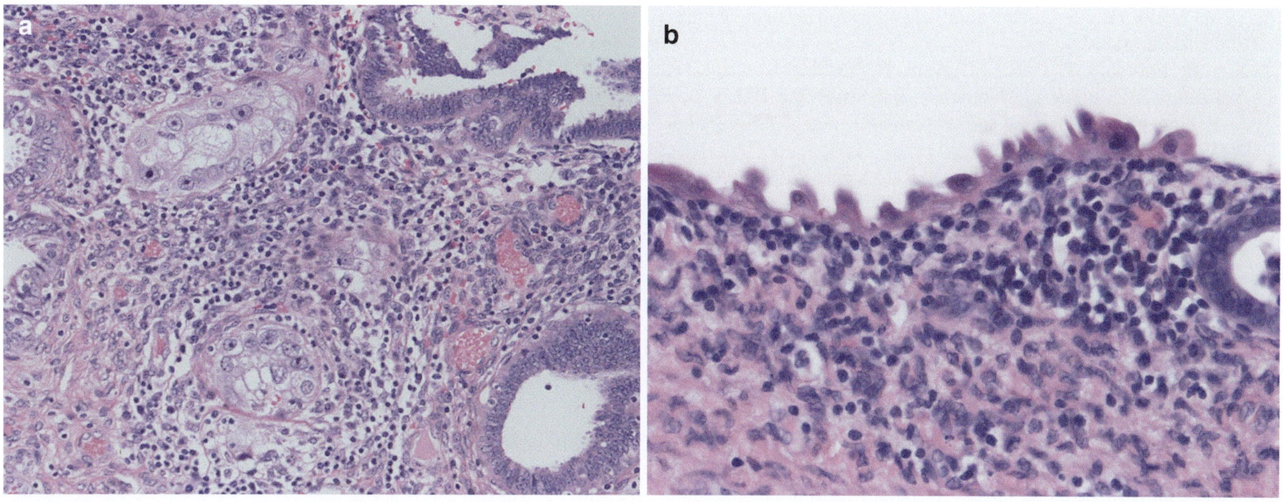

Fig. 3.13 Putative precursor lesion of clear cell carcinoma. (**a**) Epithelial cells with clear cytoplasm and marked cellular atypia proliferate in preexisting glands. (**b**) Hobnail cells with nuclear atypia proliferate on the surface of endometrium. There was clear cell carcinoma in other areas of this endometrium

prised of clear or hobnail cells with nuclear atypia in the uteri of clear cell carcinoma patients [39]. Nuclear atypia of this lesion is intermediate between background benign endometrium and full-blown clear cell carcinoma. In addition, they showed that such lesions are observed exclusively in association with pure or mixed carcinomas with a clear cell carcinoma component. They designated this type of lesion as a "putative proliferative lesion (PPL)" (Fig. 3.13). PPLs of clear cell carcinoma were identified with an average of 2.5 foci per case. Immunohistochemically, p53 expression in PPLs is not constant, and the average of Ki-67 index is 35%. PPLs show decreased expression of ER and PgR. Although morphological analysis suggests that PPLs are a precursor of clear cell carcinoma, further molecular and clinical studies are necessary to confirm this hypothesis.

Differential diagnosis of clear cell PPLs includes clear cell or hobnail metaplasia and the Arias-Stella reaction. Clear cell and hobnail metaplasia lack mitotic figures and nuclear atypia. The Arias-Stella reaction shows clear cell change of the epithelium and nuclear atypia. Clinical information of pregnancy or hormonal therapy helps differential diagnosis. Moreover, as the Arias-Stella reaction lacks p53 overexpression and a high proliferation index in contrast to PPLs, IHC of p53 and Ki-67 help this differential diagnosis [40].

References

1. Bokhman JV. Two pathogenetic types of endometrial carcinoma. Gynecol Oncol. 1983;15:10–7.
2. Kurman RJ, Kaminski PF, Norris HJ. The behavior of endometrial hyperplasia. A long-term study of "untreated" hyperplasia in 170 patients. Cancer. 1985;56:403–12.
3. Bergeron C, Nogales FF, Masseroli M, Abeler V, Duvillard P, Müller-Holzner E, Pickartz H, Wells M. A multicentric European study testing the reproducibility of the WHO classification of endometrial hyperplasia with a proposal of a simplified working classification for biopsy and curettage specimens. Am J Surg Pathol. 1999;23:1102–8.
4. Zaino R, Carineli SG, Ellenson LH, Eng C, Katabuchi H, Konishi I, Lax S, Matias-Guiu X, Mutter GL, Peters WA III, Sherman ME, Shih I-M, Soslow R, Stewart CJR. Epithelial tumours and precursors. In: Kurman RJ, Carcangiu ML, Herrington CS, Young RJ, editors. WHO classification of tumours of female reproductive organs. 4th ed. Lyon: International Agency for Research on Cancer; 2014. p. 125–35.
5. Silverberg SG. Problems in the differential diagnosis of endometrial hyperplasia and carcinoma. Mod Pathol. 2000;13:309–27.
6. Kendall BS, Ronnett BM, Isacson C, Cho KR, Hedrick L, Diener-West M, Kurman RJ. Reproducibility of the diagnosis of endometrial hyperplasia, atypical hyperplasia, and well-differentiated carcinoma. Am J Surg Pathol. 1998;22:1012–9.
7. Trimble CL, Kauderer J, Zaino R, Silverberg S, Lim PC, Burke JJ II, Alberts D, Curtin J. Concurrent endometrial carcinoma in women with a biopsy diagnosis of atypical endometrial hyperplasia: a Gynecologic Oncology Group study. Cancer. 2006;106:812–9.
8. Mutter GL. Endometrial intraepithelial neoplasia (EIN): will it bring order to chaos? The Endometrial Collaborative Group. Gynecol Oncol. 2000;76:287–90.
9. Hecht JL, Ince TA, Baak JP, Baker HE, Ogden MW, Mutter GL. Prediction of endometrial carcinoma by subjective endometrial intraepithelial neoplasia diagnosis. Mod Pathol. 2005;18:324–30.
10. Rakha E, Wong SC, Soomro I, Chaudry Z, Sharma A, Deen S, Chan S, Abu J, Nunns D, Williamson K, McGregor A, Hammond R, Brown L. Clinical outcome of atypical endometrial hyperplasia diagnosed on an endometrial biopsy: institutional experience and review of literature. Am J Surg Pathol. 2012;36:1683–90. https://doi.org/10.1097/PAS.0b013e31825dd4ff.
11. Baak JP, Mutter GL, Robboy S, van Diest PJ, Uyterlinde AM, Orbo A, Palazzo J, Fiane B, Løvslett K, Burger C, Voorhorst F, Verheijen RH. The molecular genetics and morphometry-based endometrial intraepithelial neoplasia classification system predicts disease progression in endometrial hyperplasia more accurately than the

1994 World Health Organization classification system. Cancer. 2005;103:2304–12.
12. Sun H, Enomoto T, Fujita M, Wada H, Yoshino K, Ozaki K, Nakamura T, Murata Y. Mutational analysis of the PTEN gene in endometrial carcinoma and hyperplasia. Am J Clin Pathol. 2001;115:32–8.
13. Hayes MP, Wang H, Espinal-Witter R, Douglas W, Solomon GJ, Baker SJ, Ellenson LH. PIK3CA and PTEN mutations in uterine endometrioid carcinoma and complex atypical hyperplasia. Clin Cancer Res. 2006;12(20 Pt 1):5932–5.
14. Mutter GL, Ince TA, Baak JPA, Kust G, Zhou X, Eng C. Molecular identification of latent precancers in histologically normal endometrium. Cancer Res. 2001;61:4311–4.
15. Berg A, Hoivik EA, Mjøs S, Holst F, Werner HM, Tangen IL, Taylor-Weiner A, Gibson WJ, Kusonmano K, Wik E, Trovik J, Halle MK, Øyan AM, Kalland KH, Cherniack AD, Beroukhim R, Stefansson I, Mills GB, Krakstad C, Salvesen HB. Molecular profiling of endometrial carcinoma precursor, primary and metastatic lesions suggests different targets for treatment in obese compared to non-obese patients. Oncotarget. 2015;6:1327–39. https://doi.org/10.18632/oncotarget.2675.
16. Konopka B, Janiec-Jankowska A, Kwiatkowska E, Najmoła U, Bidziński M, Olszewski W, Goluda C. PIK3CA mutations and amplification in endometrioid endometrial carcinomas: relation to other genetic defects and clinicopathologic status of the tumors. Hum Pathol. 2011;42:1710–9. https://doi.org/10.1016/j.humpath.2010.01.030.
17. Mutter GL, Wada H, Faquin WC, Enomoto T. K-ras mutations appear in the premalignant phase of both microsatellite stable and unstable endometrial carcinogenesis. Mol Pathol. 1999;52:257–62.
18. Zauber P, Denehy TR, Taylor RR, Ongcapin EH, Marotta S, Sabbath-Solitare M. Strong correlation between molecular changes in endometrial carcinomas and concomitant hyperplasia. Int J Gynecol Cancer. 2015;25:863–8. https://doi.org/10.1097/IGC.0000000000000421.
19. Saegusa M, Hashimura M, Yoshida T, Okayasu I. β- catenin mutations and aberrant nuclear expression during endometrial tumorigenesis. Br J Cancer. 2001;84:209–17.
20. Moreno-Bueno G, Hardisson D, Sarrió D, Sánchez C, Cassia R, Prat J, Herman JG, Esteller M, Matías-Guiu X, Palacios J. Abnormalities of E- and P-cadherin and catenin (beta-, gamma-catenin, and p120ctn) expression in endometrial cancer and endometrial atypical hyperplasia. J Pathol. 2003;199:471–8.
21. Wiegand KC, Lee AF, Al-Agha OM, Chow C, Kalloger SE, Scott DW, Steidl C, Wiseman SM, Gascoyne RD, Gilks B, Huntsman DG. Loss of BAF250a (ARID1A) is frequent in high-grade endometrial carcinomas. J Pathol. 2011;224:328–33. https://doi.org/10.1002/path.2911.
22. Werner HM, Berg A, Wik E, Birkeland E, Krakstad C, Kusonmano K, Petersen K, Kalland KH, Oyan AM, Akslen LA, Trovik J, Salvesen HB. ARID1A loss is prevalent in endometrial hyperplasia with atypia and low-grade endometrioid carcinomas. Mod Pathol. 2013;26:428–34. https://doi.org/10.1038/modpathol.2012.174.
23. Mao TL, Ardighieri L, Ayhan A, Kuo KT, Wu CH, Wang TL, Shih IM. Loss of ARID1A expression correlates with stages of tumor progression in uterine endometrioid carcinoma. Am J Surg Pathol. 2013;37:1342–8. https://doi.org/10.1097/PAS.0b013e3182889dc3.
24. Cohn DE, Mutch DG, Herzog TJ, Rader JS, Dintzis SM, Gersell DJ, Todd CR, Goodfellow PJ. Genotypic and phenotypic progression in endometrial tumorigenesis: determining when defects in DNA mismatch repair and KRAS2 occur. Genes Chromosomes Cancer. 2001;32:295–301.
25. Han SJ, Kim MK. Clinical significance of mismatch repair genes immunohistochemical expression of complex endometrial hyperplasia. Obstet Gynecol Sci. 2015;58:106–11. https://doi.org/10.5468/ogs.2015.58.2.106.
26. Kohler MF, Nishii H, Humphrey PA, Saski H, Marks J, Bast RC, Clarke-Pearson DL, Boyd J, Berchuck A. Mutation of the p53 tumor-suppressor gene is not a feature of endometrial hyperplasias. Am J Obstet Gynecol. 1993;169:690–4.
27. Kurman RJ, Norris HJ. Evaluation of criteria for distinguishing atypical endometrial hyperplasia from well-differentiated carcinoma. Cancer. 1982;49:2547–59.
28. Ambros RA, Sherman ME, Zahn CM, Bitterman P, Kurman RJ. Endometrial intraepithelial carcinoma: a distinctive lesion specifically associated with tumors displaying serous differentiation. Hum Pathol. 1995;26:1260–7.
29. Soslow RA, Pirog E, Isacson C. Endometrial intraepithelial carcinoma with associated peritoneal carcinomatosis. Am J Surg Pathol. 2000;24:726–32.
30. Tashiro H, Isacson C, Levine R, Kurman RJ, Cho KR, Hedrick L. p53 gene mutations are common in uterine serous carcinoma and occur early in their pathogenesis. Am J Pathol. 1997;150:177–85.
31. Zheng W, Yi X, Fadare O, Liang SX, Martel M, Schwartz PE, Jiang Z. The oncofetal protein IMP3: a novel biomarker for endometrial serous carcinoma. Am J Surg Pathol. 2008;32:304–15.
32. Lee Y, Miron A, Drapkin R, Nucci MR, Medeiros F, Saleemuddin A, Garber J, Birch C, Mou H, Gordon RW, Cramer DW, McKeon FD, Crum CP. A candidate precursor to serous carcinoma that originates in the distal fallopian tube. J Pathol. 2007;211:26–35.
33. Jarboe EA, Pizer ES, Miron A, Monte N, Mutter GL, Crum CP. Evidence for a latent precursor (p53 signature) that may precede serous endometrial intraepithelial carcinoma. Mod Pathol. 2009;22:345–50.
34. Nguyen TT, Hachisuga T, Urabe R, Kurita T, Kagami S, Kawagoe T, Shimajiri S, Nabeshima K. Significance of p53 expression in background endometrium in endometrial carcinoma. Virchows Arch. 2015;466:695–702.
35. Zhang X, Liang SX, Jia L, Chen N, Fadare O, Schwartz PE, Kong B, Zheng W. Molecular identification of "latent precancers" for endometrial serous carcinoma in benign-appearing endometrium. Am J Pathol. 2009;174(6):2000.
36. Zheng W, Liang SX, Yu H, Rutherford T, Chambers SK, Schwartz PE. Endometrial glandular dysplasia: a newly defined precursor lesion of uterine papillary serous carcinoma. Part I: morphologic features. Int J Surg Pathol. 2004;12:207–23.
37. Liang SX, Chambers SK, Cheng L, Zhang S, Zhou Y, Zheng W. Endometrial glandular dysplasia: a putative precursor lesion of uterine papillary serous carcinoma. Part II: molecular features. Int J Surg Pathol. 2004;12:319–31.
38. Lax SF, Pizer ES, Ronnett BM, Kurman RJ. Clear cell carcinoma of the endometrium is characterized by a distinctive profile of p53, Ki-67, estrogen, and progesterone receptor expression. Hum Pathol. 1998;29:551–8.
39. Fadare O, Liang SX, Ulukus EC, Chambers SK, Zheng W. Precursors of endometrial clear cell carcinoma. Am J Surg Pathol. 2006;30:1519–30.
40. Vang R, Barner R, Wheeler DT, et al. Immunohistochemical staining for Ki-67 and p53 helps distinguish endometrial Arias-Stella reaction from high-grade carcinoma, including clear cell carcinoma. Int J Gynecol Pathol. 2004;23:223–33.

Current Concept of Precancerous and Early Stage of Serous Ovarian Carcinoma

4

Takako Kiyokawa and Masami Iwamoto

Abstract

Two types of ovarian serous carcinomas are recognized including high-grade (HGSC) and low-grade serous carcinoma (LGSC). These fundamentally differ in terms of histology, phenotype, underlying genetics, carcinogenetic mechanisms, and biological behavior. The vast majority of them are HGSC.

Recent evidence strongly suggests most cases considered as ovarian HGSC according to the classical definition are secondary involvement of tubal HGSC, either in the form of non-invasive or invasive HGSC. Serous tubal intraepithelial carcinoma (STIC) is a non-invasive tubal HGSC and is detected mostly at the fimbriated end. Tumor protein (TP)53 mutations are present in most HGSC cases and BRCA network dysregulation in 50%. More than 80% of HGSC patients present with advanced stage disease (Stage III/IV) . HGSC patients have poor prognosis: although most HGSC responds to platinum/taxol chemotherapy after debulking surgery, the majority of cases show recurrence leading to death.

LGSC often coexists with and is thought to arise from serous borderline tumor. About 40%–60% of LGSC harbor somatic mutations in KRAS and BRAF. TP53 or BRCA mutation is rare in LGSC. LGSC confined to the ovary has excellent prognosis with surgical therapy alone; however, invasive LGSC is less responsive to current platinumbased chemotherapy regimens than HGSC.

Keywords

Ovarian tumor · Serous carcinoma · Serous borderline tumor · Serous tubal intraepithelial carcinoma

T. Kiyokawa (✉) · M. Iwamoto
Department of Pathology, The Jikei University School of Medicine, Tokyo, Japan
e-mail: kiyokawa@jikei.ac.jp

4.1 General Concept of Ovarian Serous Carcinoma (SC)

Serous tumors are defined as epithelial neoplasia with tubal differentiation. In both serous adenoma and serous borderline tumors (SBTs), tumor cells simulate fallopian tube epithelial cells—namely, ciliated, peg, and secretory cells. Although tumor cells in SC—an invasive counterpart of serous tumors—do not morphologically resemble epithelial cells of the normal fallopian tube, they share phenotypic features with tubal secretory cells [1].

About 90% of all ovarian malignancies are of the epithelial type, which includes high-grade (HG) SC, low-grade (LG) SC, endometrioid carcinoma, clear cell carcinoma, and mucinous carcinoma, among others. High-grade SC accounts for 60–80% of cases of epithelial-type malignancies in western countries [2] and 38% of those in Japan, which has a much higher incidence of clear cell carcinoma (25%, higher than in western countries) [3].

Two types of ovarian SC are recognized based on recent evidence, including high- and low-grade types [4]. These fundamentally differ in terms of histology, phenotype, underlying genetics, carcinogenetic mechanisms, and biological behavior. Neither tumor type has been further graded histologically. The vast majority of SCs (approximately 95%) are of high grade.

4.2 HGSC

HGSC is histologically characterized by invasive adenocarcinoma with high-grade tumor cells (Figs. 4.1 and 4.2) that have an eosinophilic cytoplasm, enlarged nuclei of variable shape and size (nuclear pleomorphism), irregularly distributed nuclear chromatin, and prominent nucleoli. Multinucleated tumor cells are also common. Mitosis proceeds at a high rate, with usually >13 mitoses detected per 10 high-power fields (HPFs) [5]. The cells typically form irregular or closely packed papillae or solid nests with or without slit-like spaces, but glandular or cribriform patterns are also

T. Moriya (ed.), *Pathology of Female Cancers*, https://doi.org/10.1007/978-981-10-8606-9_4

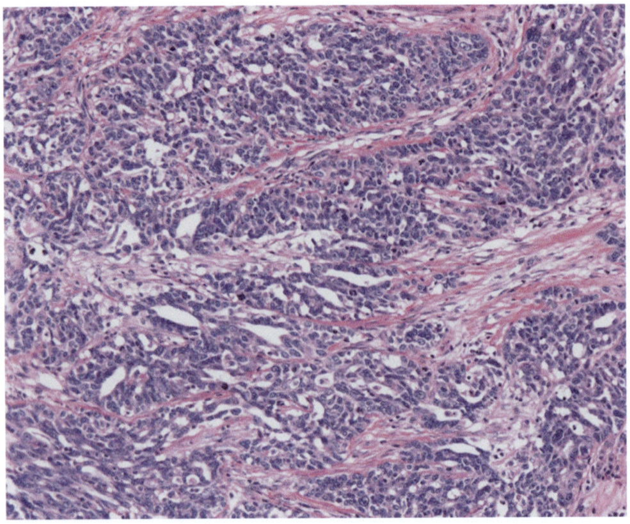

Fig. 4.1 High-grade serous carcinoma. Tumor cells are arranged in nests with slit-like spaces or fused glands and are infiltrating in the stroma

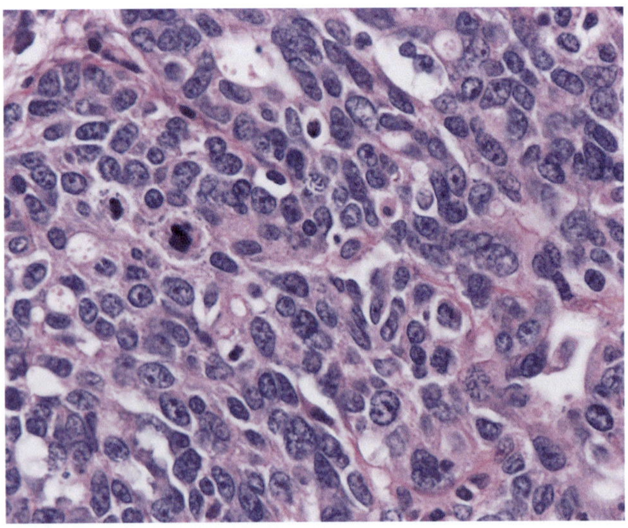

Fig. 4.2 High-grade serous carcinoma. Tumor cells have eosinophilic cytoplasm and enlarged nuclei of variable shape and size. Prominent nucleoli and atypical mitosis are also seen

observed. Cases previously classified as ovarian transitional cell carcinoma are now thought to represent a variant of HGSC and rarely of endometrioid carcinoma [6–8]. Women with *breast cancer* (*BRC*)*A1/2* germline mutations have a 30–70% risk of developing ovarian cancer by the age of 70 [9] and also have increased risk of developing breast cancer; such cases are designated as hereditary breast and ovarian cancer (HBOC). Most of these ovarian cancers are of the high-grade serous type. One study described the characteristic histological features of HGSC associated with HBOC, including solid, pseudoendometrioid, and transitional cell carcinoma-like morphology (referred to as SET features); necrosis; and prominent lymphocytic infiltration [10]. Immunohistochemically, tumor cells often exhibit aberrant p53 expression (strong and diffuse or completely absent staining) and positivity for Wilms tumor (WT)-1, $p16^{Ink4a}$ (cyclin-dependent kinase inhibitor 2A), and estrogen receptor (ER) and are almost always diffusely positive for paired box gene (PAX) 8 [11, 12].

HGSC tends to occur in postmenopausal women, typically in those in their 6th and 7th decades, with a mean age of 63 years old. More than 80% of patients present with advanced-stage disease (stage III/IV), with few cases confined to the ovaries (<10%); serum CA-125 is usually elevated in these patients, with a median value in the range of 200–1000 U/mL [13]. HGSC patients have poor prognosis, with 5- and 10-year survival rates of 9%–49% and 13%–16%, respectively [5, 14–16]. Although most HGSC responds to platinum/taxol chemotherapy after debulking surgery, the majority of cases show recurrence leading to death. The most important prognostic factor for patients is disease stage; for advanced-stage cases, the amount of residual tumor after debulking and staging is the major determinant of prognosis, with patients in whom complete resection is achieved showing a significantly better outcome [17].

Tumor protein (*TP*)*53* mutations are present in most HGSC cases. Although germline and somatic *BRCA1/2* mutations occur at a rate of 15–20%, dysregulation of the *BRCA* network is more widespread (50%) [2, 18, 19]. Recent studies by The Cancer Genome Atlas project revealed that HGSCs could be further classified into mesenchymal, immunoreactive, proliferative, and differentiated subtypes [19, 20]. This was confirmed in an Australian population, and in both studies, the mesenchymal and immunoreactive types had poor and favorable prognosis, respectively. Another study described novel histopathological HGSC subtypes according to gene expression, prognosis, and sensitivity to specific chemotherapeutic agents [21], although this classification has not yet been validated by other groups.

The origin and pathogenesis of HGSC have been long debated. It was previously thought to arise from ovarian surface epithelium or an epithelial inclusion cyst as a result of ovulation, without a precursor lesion [22]. However, recent evidence strongly suggests an origin in the fallopian tube in most cases where the metastatic ovarian mass is clinically dominant [1, 23–25]. This was first noted in a comprehensive examination of ovaries and fallopian tubes of risk-reducing salpingo-oophorectomy (RRSO) specimens from women with *BRCA1/2* germline mutations and/or those with a family history of ovarian cancer, which revealed that non-invasive or minimally invasive SC was much more common in the fallopian tubes—usually at the fimbriated end—than in the ovary [23, 26–28]. This shifted the focus to the fallopian tubes, which had previously been considered as an unusual site for primary carcinoma. The earliest evidence of HGSC in RRSO specimens was intramucosal lesions known as serous tubal intraepithelial carcinoma (STIC) (see below) [23, 25]. The sectioning and extensively examining the fimbria (SEE-FIM) protocol has been developed for detailed systematic examination of the fallopian tubes [24]. SEE-FIM entails fixation of the entire tube and serial longitudinal sectioning of the distal 2 cm of the fimbriated end, followed by transverse sectioning

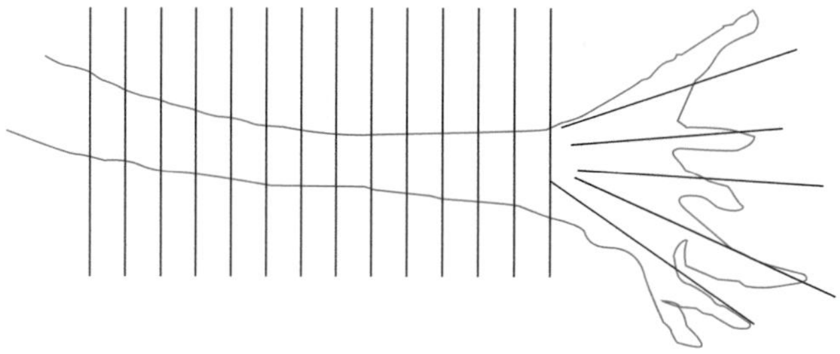

Fig. 4.3 Protocol for sectioning and extensively examining the fimbriated end (SEE-FIM) of the fallopian tube [24]. The distal 2 cm of the fimbriated end of the fallopian tube is serially and longitudinally sectioned, and the remaining are sectioned every 2–3 mm

of every 2–3 mm of the remaining tissue (Fig. 4.3). Using this protocol, STICs were detected in 40–60% of women with HGSC with or without *BRCA* germline mutations that would have been considered primary in the ovary (or peritoneum) according to the classical criteria [25, 29–31]. In up to 20% of HGSC patients, the fallopian tube (or at least, its fimbriated end) is completely obliterated by adnexal tumors in the ipsilateral ovary. These cases are considered to be primary fallopian tube carcinoma even in the absence of STIC. The following lines of evidence further support the fallopian tube as the site of origin and STIC as the precursor lesion of HGSC.

1. The majority of incidentally detected organ-confined HGSCs in *BRCA*-unrelated patients are located in the unilateral fallopian tube mucosa only—especially at the fimbriated end—without ovarian involvement [32].
2. STICs associated with advanced-stage HGSC harbor identical *TP53* mutations in the disseminated tumor [33, 34], indicating that they are clonal.
3. Comparison of telomere length in matched STIC and ovarian tumor pairs suggests that the former precedes the latter [35].
4. Centrosome amplification is greater in ovarian tumor samples than in paired STICs [36], indicating that the latter are the earlier or precursor lesion.
5. In patients with synchronous tubal and ovarian HGSC involvement, bilateral ovarian involvement is more frequently observed than bilateral tubal involvement [37].

In a subset of HGSC patients, extensive histological examination fails to demonstrate tubal HGSC or STIC. It has been suggested that some cases of HGSC with normal fallopian tubes arise from benign epithelial cells of tubal origin that became implanted in the ovaries at ovulation. SBTs with or without micropapillary patterns are rarely precursors of HGSC and typically do not recur as HGSC.

There is potential for confusion in establishing the primary site of HGSC due to the tubal origin of most HGSCs mentioned above. A revised International Federation of Gynecology and Obstetrics (FIGO) staging system was introduced in 2014 to encompass tumors arising in the ovary, fallopian tube, and peritoneum and to address the absence of specific internationally agreed guidelines for assigning the primary site of HGSCs. The FIGO system recommends that the primary site (i.e., ovary, fallopian tube, or peritoneum) be designated where possible; cases where this is not possible are classified as "undesignated" [38]. The World Health Organization (WHO) classification revised in 2014 recommends that the professional judgment be exercised when designating a lesion site as primary. A recent study proposed a new practical guideline for establishing the primary site of HGSCs that is applicable to both chemo-naïve and post-chemotherapy cases, and this has also been adopted for recommendation in the histopathology reporting guide by the International Collaboration on Cancer Reporting (ICCR) [37, 39, 40] (Table 4.1): for example, any

Table 4.1 Suggestions for assigning site of origin [39]

1. The fallopian tubes, or at least their fimbriated ends, should be totally sampled in all cases of HGSC by a SEE-FIM-like protocol to avoid missing this important site of disease
2. The presence of STIC without invasion or extratubal spread should be staged as FIGO stage IA tubal carcinoma, but with an annotation that there is no invasive carcinoma
3. Cases with only STIC, ovarian surface involvement or parenchymal involvement not exceeding 5 mm, and widespread peritoneal involvement, which would be categorized traditionally as primary peritoneal carcinoma, should be classified as tubal primaries
4. Cases with invasive HGSC located within the mucosa of the fallopian tube, including its fimbriated end, with or without STIC in any portion of the fallopian tube and with no, minimal or even substantial ovarian involvement, should be categorized as tubal primaries
5. Cases in which the fallopian tube is not identifiable, having presumably been overgrown by the ipsilateral adnexal mass, or the distal end of the fallopian tube is incorporated into a large tubo-ovarian mass should also be diagnosed as tubal primaries. It is emphasized that a careful effort must be made to identify the tube in all cases
6. Cases with dominant ovarian mass(es) and identifiable fallopian tubes with STIC should be classified as tubal primaries
7. Cases with dominant ovarian mass(es) and identifiable fallopian tubes without STIC should be classified as ovarian primaries
8. Cases should be categorized as primary peritoneal carcinoma by the conventional criteria below and only after complete examination of the fallopian tubes (including the non-fimbrial portions) has excluded the presence of STIC or a small HGSC: • Both ovaries must be normal in size or enlarged by a benign process • The involvement in the extra-ovarian sites must be greater than the involvement on the surface of either ovary • The ovarian tumor involvement must be nonexistent, confined to the ovarian surface without stromal invasion, or involve the cortical stroma with tumor size less than 5 × 5 mm
9. All cases classified as 'undesignated' for FIGO staging purposes should be further described as 'tubo-ovarian' or 'tubal/ovarian' to distinguish them from serous carcinoma originating in the uterus. Using our suggestions, these should represent a small proportion of HGSC.
10. Cases with unilateral or bilateral HGSC in the ovary and/or STIC or HGSC in the tube but with an endometrial serous intraepithelial or invasive carcinoma should be evaluated carefully for an endometrial versus a tubo-ovarian primary (WT-1 staining may be of value); a majority of such cases will represent adnexal metastases from an endometrial serous carcinoma

case exhibiting STIC or tubal intramucosal involvement would be classified as tubal primary. According to this guideline, the fallopian tubes—or at least their fimbriated ends—must be entirely sampled in all cases of HGSC with a SEE-FIM-like protocol to avoid overlooking this important site of disease. This group also proposed that STIC be considered as stage Ia, since there was no solid basis for supposing that STIC detected as an incidental finding is a bona fide in situ disease, and complete staging of such cases may reveal them as advanced stage [37]. Uniform staging and site assignment will enable prospective data collection. It should be noted that this new proposal does not necessarily follow the approach recommended by the FIGO committee. For example, a case of a tumor limited to one ovary and STIC without evidence of direct extension from the latter to the former would be classified as tubal primary according to the new guideline but as stage IA ovarian carcinoma with STIC by the FIGO committee [41].

Most cases considered as ovarian HGSC according to the classical definition show secondary involvement of tubal HGSC (either in the form of STIC or invasive HGSC), with STIC as the precursor lesion. Based on these observations, fallopian tubes are removed at the time of hysterectomy or tubal ligation, a procedure referred to as opportunistic salpingectomy, which is considered a promising approach for preventing HGSC [42–45].

4.3 STIC

STIC is defined as a non-invasive SC of the fallopian tube that is histologically characterized by proliferation of malignant cells in the tubal epithelium (Figs. 4.4 and 4.5). Tumor cells in STIC are identical to those in HGSC, showing an elevated nuclear/cytoplasmic ratio with more rounded nuclei,

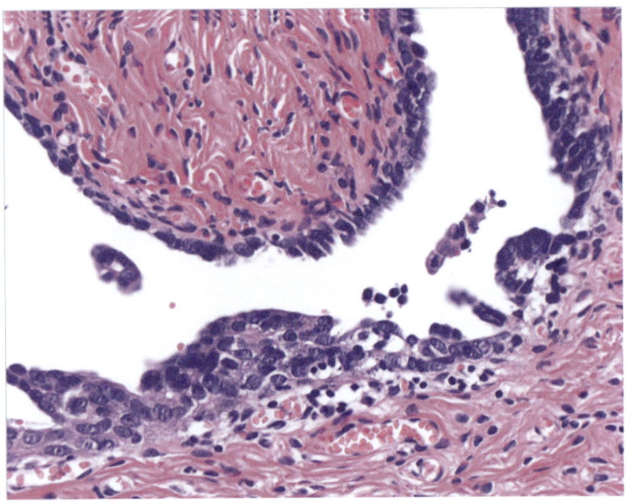

Fig. 4.4 Serous tubal intraepithelial carcinoma (STIC). Multilayered highly atypical cells are replacing the tubal epithelium (lower half and right). Note the absence of ciliated cells and loss of polarity, and some cells are shedding into the tubal lumen

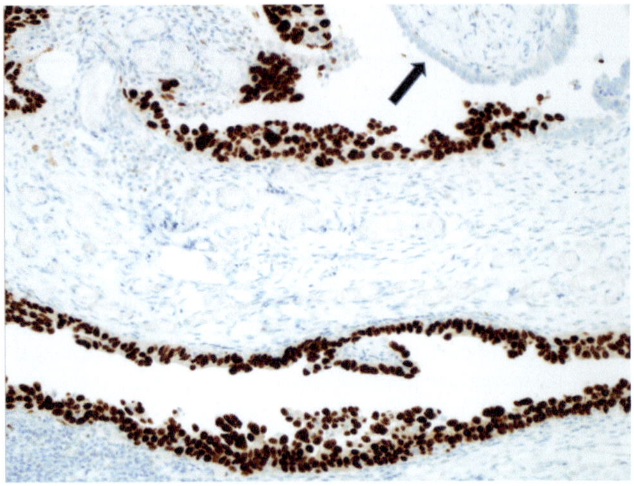

Fig. 4.5 Serous tubal intraepithelial carcinoma (STIC), p53 immunohistochemistry. Cells of STIC are diffusely stained for p53, whereas normal tubal epithelia (arrow) are not

nuclear hyperchromasia and pleomorphism, prominent nucleoli, mitotic figures, absence of ciliated cells, and loss of polarity. They are typically multilayered and discohesive and are frequently shed into the tubal lumen. Criteria for distinguishing exuberant non-invasive HGSC from large STIC have yet to be defined. STIC is grossly invisible and is detected throughout the distal tube, mostly at the fimbriated end, and can therefore be easily missed or underestimated without employing the SEE-FIM protocol or at least examining serial longitudinal sections of the fimbriated end of resected fallopian tubes. Immunohistochemically, STIC cells show aberrant expression of p53 (usually strong and diffuse and—less commonly—completely negative staining). The Ki-67 index is markedly elevated, ranging from 40 to 95% (mean, 72%), although there are no specific cutoff values as a stand-alone parameter to distinguish STIC from other intraepithelial changes [46]. p16, ER, and WT-1 may also be expressed [47]. Although in most of cases STIC can be successfully diagnosed by morphology alone, p53 and Ki-67 immunohistochemistry combined with morphology has shown to improve the reproducibility of STIC vs. non-STIC diagnoses [48, 49]. STIC cells are also immunopositive for the tubal secretory cell markers HMFG2 and Stathmin 1 [1, 50] and for gamma-H2AX, suggesting double-stranded DNA damage [51].

It should be noted that although rare, secondary involvement of the fallopian tube mucosa can obfuscate diagnosis. Endometrial SC may exhibit transtubal spread; in such cases, mucosal involvement of the fallopian tube may be indistinguishable from STIC based on morphology alone. WT-1 negativity in both tubal and endometrial lesions suggests a primary site in the endometrium, since WT-1 is usually negative in endometrial SC and diffusely positive in non-uterine HGSC [32, 52]. Non-gynecologic primary tumors may also involve tubal mucosa—usually at the fimbriated end—that morphologically resemble STIC. In these cases, clinical correlation as well as anatomical distribution of the disease must be considered, with appropriate use of immunohistochemistry required for correct diagnosis [53, 54].

Early studies of tubal mucosa identified small foci composed of at least 12 consecutive non-ciliated (i.e., secretory) cells showing strong and diffuse p53 immunoreactivity but with histologically benign appearance. These were abundant in the fimbriated end of the tube and have been designated as p53 signatures [1, 24]. As in STIC, most of the foci showed immunohistochemical evidence of double-stranded DNA damage [1, 51]. They were more frequent and multifocal in tubes with STIC, with which they were possibly continuous [1]. About 57% of p53 signatures have *TP53* mutations, although the Ki-67 index is low (mean, 3%) [2], and they are detected in women with and without *BRCA* mutations at the same frequency (10%–38% vs. 17%–33%). Thus, p53 signatures probably represent early clonal expansion without neoplastic proliferation, with *TP53* mutation being an early event in foci leading to STIC [2]. It is possible that STIC development is promoted by germline *BRCA1* mutation [2, 55]. Several terms have been proposed for lesions that fall between p53 signatures and STIC, including tubal intraepithelial lesions in transition, serous tubal epithelial proliferation, serous tubal intraepithelial lesions, serous tubal intraepithelial lesions of uncertain significance, and tubal epithelial atypia [46].

The incidence of STIC in RRSO specimens from women with *BRCA* mutation is variable, ranging from 1 to 7% (mean, 5.2%) [56, 57]. Since STIC alone is thought to be associated with a favorable prognosis with rare cases of recurrence, surgical staging has been deemed unnecessary for these patients when peritoneal cytology is negative [58]. On the other hand, peritoneal washing cytology is routinely recommended at RRSO for high-risk patients, since the high incidence of positive peritoneal cytology in STIC patients may provide important prognostic information [56, 57]. Only a few studies have reported the incidence of STIC in low-risk women undergoing salpingectomy for benign reasons [46, 59]. Given that STIC is presumed to be present for a relatively short time before progressing to metastasis [60] and only approximately 1% of women will develop HGSC during their lifetime, it is reasonable to suppose that <1% of salpingectomy specimens from low-risk patients harbor STIC [32].

4.4 LGSC

Invasive LGSC is rare, comprising only about 5% of SC cases. Histologically, LGSC is characterized by serous tumors composed of uniform tumor cells infiltrating into the stroma that are ≥5 mm (Figs. 4.6 and 4.7). LGSC cell nuclei

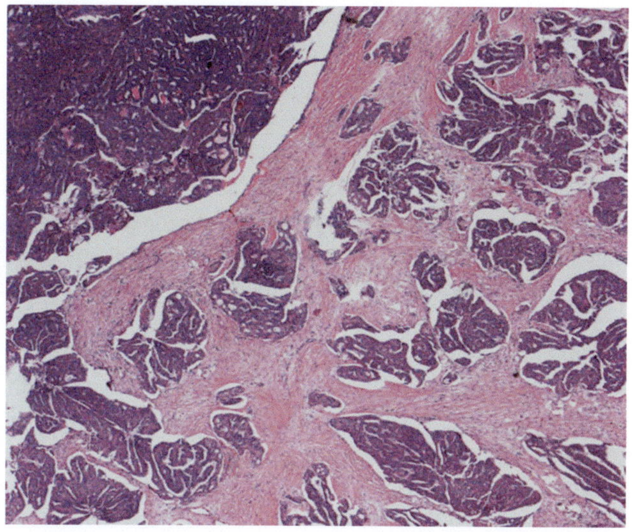

Fig. 4.6 Low-grade serous carcinoma. Tumor cells show various patterns and infiltrating in the fibrous stroma. Cleft-like spaces are found surrounding papillary structures or clusters of cells

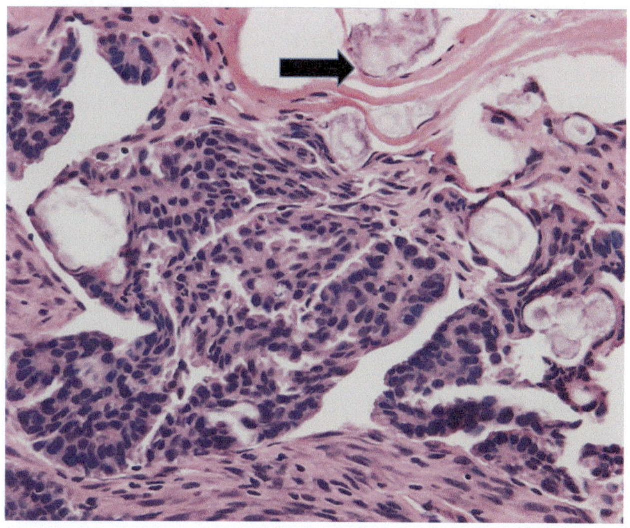

Fig. 4.7 Low-grade serous carcinoma. Small and uniform tumor cells form irregular nests or papillae and are infiltrating in the stroma. Calcification is prominent (arrow) and stroma is fibrous

are small and oval or round; the nuclear chromatin is uniform or only slightly irregular, and mitotic activity is <13/10 HPFs (mean, 4/10 HPFs). Their architectural patterns are variable. Micropapillae or irregular small nests are most common, but glands, macropapillae, and single cells are also observed. Cleft-like or non-epithelial-lined spaces typically surround papillary structures or cell clusters, and a desmoplastic reaction may or may not be present. Necrosis is rarely observed. Calcification—including psammoma bodies—is much more frequent and extensive than in HGSC and is often grossly recognizable. Invasive LGSC often coexists with and is thought to arise from typical SBTs with or without MP/non-invasive low-grade SC (see below).

Immunohistochemically, LGSCs are identical to SBTs except for a lower rate of progesterone receptor (PgR) expression (50% of cases) and are typically positive for PAX8, WT-1, and ER, showing wild-type p53 expression while lacking diffuse p16 staining [11, 12].

LGSC patients are 5–10 years younger than HGSC patients [61], and their tumors usually have surface involvement, with only about 10% confined to the ovary at presentation [5, 62]. Progression-free and overall survival are longer in invasive LGSC patients than in those with HGSC [5, 62, 63], although some studies have shown different results [16]. LGSC confined to the ovary has excellent prognosis with surgical therapy alone; however, invasive LGSC is less responsive to current platinum-based chemotherapy regimens than HGSC [64].

About 40%–60% of invasive LGSC, MP, and SBT cases harbor somatic mutations in *KRAS* and *BRAF* and less frequently in *ERBB2* [12]; however, these are rare in high-grade tumors [61]. These three genes encode upstream regulators of mitogen-activated protein kinase (MAPK); their mutations are mutually exclusive and could result in constitutive activation of MAPK signaling, leading to uncontrolled proliferation [12, 65]. Mutations in RAS-RAF-MAPK signaling components in these tumors suggest that this pathway is a potential therapeutic target [61, 66]. SBTs and MPs appear to develop from serous cystadenomas, progressing very slowly toward invasive LGSC. Mutations in either *KRAS* or *BRAF* identical to those observed in LGSC have also been detected in cystadenomas adjacent to SBTs, but not in those unassociated with SBTs, suggesting that this is an early event in the transition from cystadenoma to SBT [67]. *TP53* or *BRCA* mutation is rare in LGSC [12].

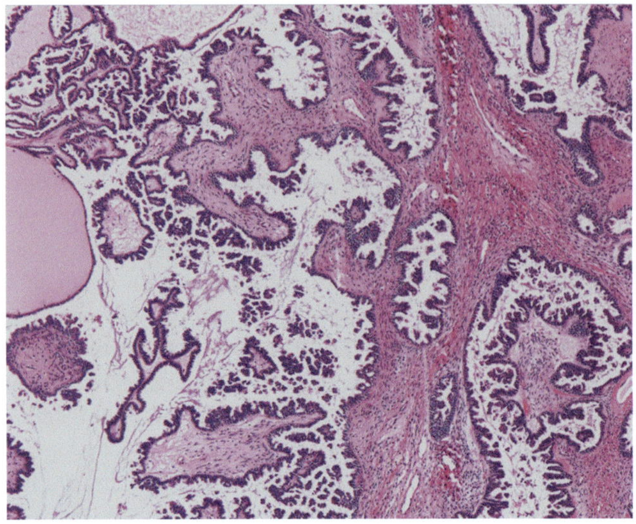

Fig. 4.8 Serous borderline tumor/atypical proliferative serous tumor. Hierarchical branching papillae terminated in detached epithelial tufts are seen

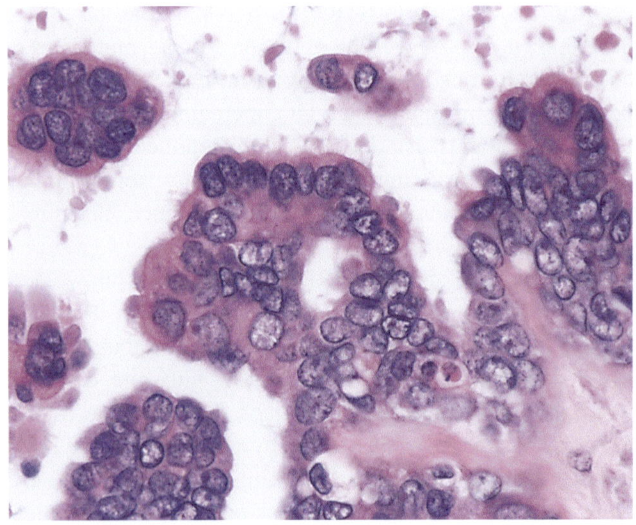

Fig. 4.9 Serous borderline tumor/atypical proliferative serous tumor. Tumor cells are stratified and are composed of admixture of ciliated and non-ciliated polygonal cells with eosinophilic cytoplasm. Nuclear atypia is moderate and mitoses are rare

4.5 SBT/Atypical Proliferative Serous Tumors and SBT/MP Variant/Non-invasive LGSC

SBT is defined as a non-invasive serous tumor with obvious epithelial proliferation and tufting. Histologically, SBTs have hierarchically branching, irregular large papillae that become progressively smaller papillae terminating in detached epithelial tufts (Fig. 4.8). The papillae are lined by epithelial cells, which are often stratified. The tumor cells are typically columnar and ciliated, and admixed with non-ciliated polygonal or hobnail cells with an eosinophilic cytoplasm (Fig. 4.9). Cells with clear cytoplasm may also be present. The nuclei show mild-to-moderate atypia and occasionally nucleoli. Classification as SBT requires an SBT component of $\geq$10% within a serous cystadenoma or cystadenofibroma. SBT can contain foci of microinvasion, which are defined as isolated or clusters of epithelial cells in the stroma that measure <5 mm along the greatest dimension [4]. Microinvasive clusters are often surrounded by retraction spaces and a fibroblast-rich stroma. The epithelial cells of these foci resemble those on the papillary surface, but tend to have an abundant eosinophilic cytoplasm and a lower Ki-67 index, underscoring their senescent nature [68]. Microinvasion is more frequently seen in SBT diagnosed during pregnancy [68]. Immunohistochemically, SBTs are usually positive for PAX8, WT-1, ER, PgR, and B cell lymphoma (bcl)-2 [69–71]; grossly, they are unilocular or oligolocular cystic tumors with or without exophytic excrescences on the ovarian surface (Fig. 4.10). Approximately one-third of SBTs are bilateral. Pelvic lymph nodes in patients with SBT may contain endosalpingiosis, individual or clusters of epithelial cells, non-invasive implants (see below), and LGSC; none of the former three types of lesion have prognostic significance [68].

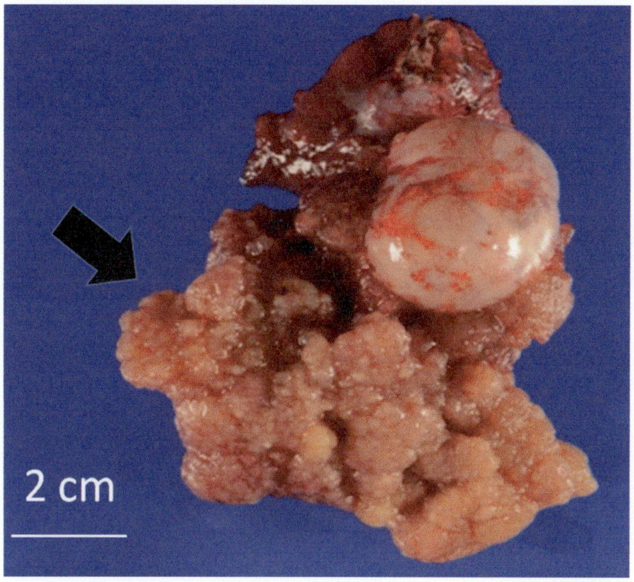

Fig. 4.10 Serous borderline tumor/atypical proliferative serous tumor. Exophytic excrescences on the ovarian surface are seen (arrow)

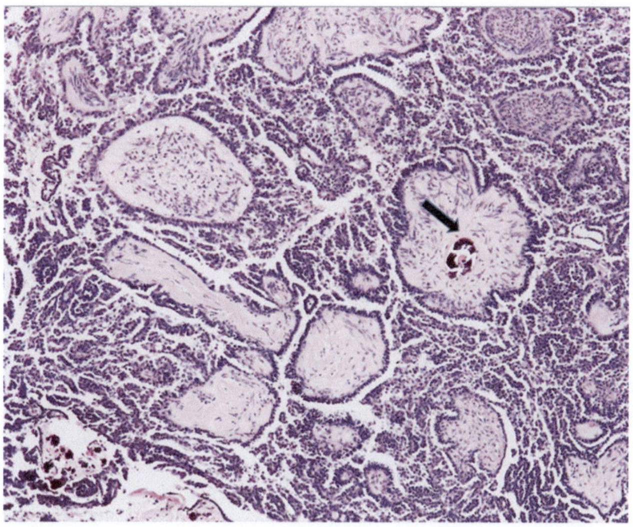

Fig. 4.11 Serous borderline tumor, micropapillary variant/non-invasive low-grade serous carcinoma. Tumor forms nonhierarchical filiform papillae without stromal invasion. Calcification is seen in the stroma (arrow)

A minority of SBTs contain micropapillary foci, which are defined as nonhierarchical filiform papillae more than five times longer than wide with minimal or absent stromal cores (Figs. 4.11 and 4.12). Cribriform or solid pattern foci may be also be present either alone or admixed with micropapillary pattern. A solid pattern results from florid cellular stratification to the extent that tumor cells fill the cystic lumen. Tumor cells in these three patterns resemble those of invasive LGSC: they are cuboidal to polygonal without cilia and have a high nuclear/cytoplasmic ratio and small, uniform, and more atypical nuclei than those of SBTs. Small but prominent cherry-red nucleoli are also often observed by

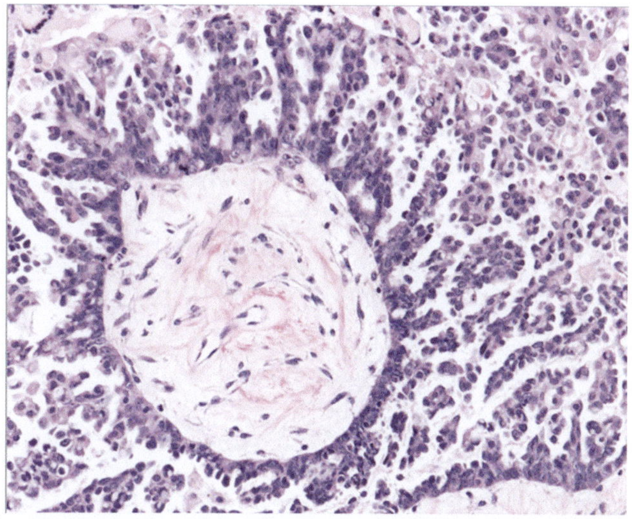

Fig. 4.12 Serous borderline tumor, micropapillary variant/non-invasive low-grade serous carcinoma. Papillae are more than five times longer than wide with minimal or absent stromal cores. Tumor cells are uniform and are resembling those of LGSC

hematoxylin and eosin staining. SBTs with at least one confluent area of micropapillary/cribriform/solid pattern measuring 5 mm in one dimension are designated as MP [4] and are thought to be the precursor lesion of invasive LGSC; those with micropapillary/cribriform/solid pattern measuring <5 mm are classified as SBT.

Approximately one-third of SBTs/MPs are associated with peritoneal implants, which were previously classified as non-invasive or invasive, with the former being most pervasive. In the WHO classification revised in 2014, non-invasive implants are designated as implants, and it is recommended that any invasive foci be labeled as peritoneal LGSC, reflecting their similar biological behaviors [4, 72, 73]. Implants/non-invasive implants are defined as proliferating serous epithelial cells confined to the peritoneal surface without infiltration of the underlying subperitoneal tissue, or it follow the omental fibrovascular septa (Figs. 4.13 and 4.14). The tumor cells are arranged in a papillary or tubular pattern or as a solid nest or single cell with or without granulation-tissue-type stromal reaction. The epithelial cells are similar to those of SBTs: they are columnar and may be ciliated, with mild-to-moderate nuclear atypia and a low rate of mitosis [61]. Peritoneal LGSC/invasive implants are characterized by extensive epithelial cells with haphazardly arranged glands, solid nests, and/or papillae accompanied by desmoplastic stroma with destructive invasion into the underlying subperitoneal tissue or omental fat. Epithelial predominance and the presence of an MP and/or a solid nesting pattern are features that can assist the diagnosis of peritoneal LGSC/invasive implants [61]. The epithelial cells are usually cuboidal or polygonal with high nuclear/cytoplasmic ratio, with small and uniform nuclei and occasional mitotic figures.

SBTs and MPs occur in the same age group (mean, 42 years) [4, 74]; they are unrelated to *BRCA* mutations [75]

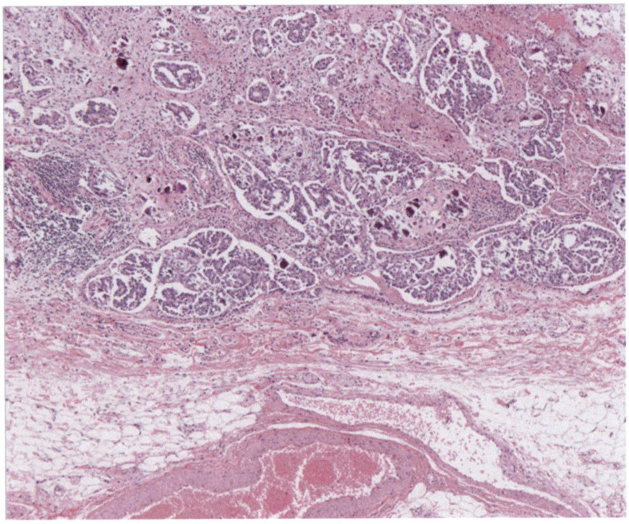

Fig. 4.13 Peritoneal implant/non-invasive implant. Proliferation of tumor cells is confined to the peritoneal surface without infiltrating the underlying subperitoneal fat

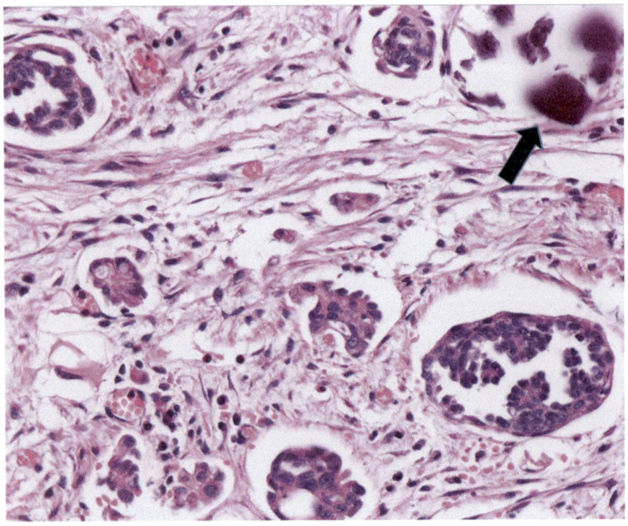

Fig. 4.14 Peritoneal implant/non-invasive implant. Tumor cells are arranged in papillary, tubular, solid nest, or single cell with granulation-tissue type stromal reaction. Calcification is also seen (arrow)

but are more often associated with a history of infertility than HGSC. SBTs are bilateral in about one-third of patients [4]. Patients with SBT confined to the ovaries (FIGO stage I) have excellent prognosis, with a disease-free survival rate of 98.2% and disease-specific survival rate of 99.5% [76]. Patients with advanced-stage SBTs have a low but definite risk of recurrence in long-term follow-ups [74]. In a meta-analysis, both MP and microinvasion were associated with higher recurrence rates (36% and 23%, respectively), but recent studies found no association between microinvasion and recurrence or survival rate [73, 76]. MPs are more frequently bilateral, have surface and peritoneal involvement, and are more often associated with stromal invasion either in the ovarian tumor or in the peritoneum on extensive sampling [61, 74, 77, 78]. Recurrence is more frequent, and progression-free survival is shorter in patients with MP than in those with typical SBT [61, 73]. Although MP alone is not an independent prognostic factor, its occurrence is a strong predictor for concurrent invasive peritoneal disease [76]. Patients with implants/non-invasive implants have excellent prognosis with a survival rate of nearly 100%. In contrast, those with peritoneal LGSC/invasive implants have shorter overall survival [71, 73–76], with a rate of 66% at 7.4 years [76]. Peritoneal LGSC/invasive implants are usually associated with MPs and implants/non-invasive implants with SBTs. It should be noted, however, that while rare, patients with SBTs or MPs who have implants/non-invasive implants may later develop progressive serous tumors and die of the disease [74, 79].

References

1. Lee Y, Miron A, Drapkin R, Nucci MR, Medeiros F, Saleemuddin A, Garber J, Birch C, Mou H, Gordon RW, Cramer DW, McKeon FD, Crum CP. A candidate precursor to serous carcinoma that originates in the distal fallopian tube. J Pathol. 2007;211:26–35.
2. Prat J. Ovarian carcinomas: five distinct diseases with different origins, genetic alterations, and clinicopathological features. Virchows Arch. 2012;460:237–49.
3. The Committee on Gynecologic Oncology, Japan Society of Obstetrics and Gynecology. Patient Annual Report for 2015. Acta Obsterica et Gynaecololgica Japonica 2017;69:1211.
4. Kurman RJ, Carcangiu ML, Herrington CS, Young RH. WHO Classification of Tumours of Female Reproductive Organs. Lyon: IARC Press; 2014.
5. Malpica A, Deavers MT, Lu K, Bodurka DC, Atkinson EN, Gershenson DM, Silva EG. Grading ovarian serous carcinoma using a two-tier system. Am J Surg Pathol. 2004;28:496–504.
6. Takeuchi T, Ohishi Y, Imamura H, Aman M, Shida K, Kobayashi H, Kato K, Oda Y. Ovarian transitional cell carcinoma represents a poorly differentiated form of high-grade serous or endometrioid adenocarcinoma. Am J Surg Pathol. 2013;37:1091–9.
7. Cuatrecasas M, Catasus L, Palacios J, Prat J. Transitional cell tumors of the ovary: a comparative clinicopathologic, immunohistochemical, and molecular genetic analysis of Brenner tumors and transitional cell carcinomas. Am J Surg Pathol. 2009;33:556–67.
8. Ali RH, Seidman JD, Luk M, Kalloger S, Gilks CB. Transitional cell carcinoma of the ovary is related to high-grade serous carcinoma and is distinct from malignant brenner tumor. Int J Gynecol Pathol. 2012;31:499–506.
9. Risch HA, McLaughlin JR, Cole DE, Rosen B, Bradley L, Fan I, Tang J, Li S, Zhang S, Shaw PA, Narod SA. Population BRCA1 and BRCA2 mutation frequencies and cancer penetrances: a kin-cohort study in Ontario, Canada. J Natl Cancer Inst. 2006;98:1694–706.
10. Soslow RA, Han G, Park KJ, Garg K, Olvera N, Spriggs DR, Kauff ND, Levine DA. Morphologic patterns associated with BRCA1 and BRCA2 genotype in ovarian carcinoma. Mod Pathol. 2012;25:625–36.
11. O'Neill CJ, McBride HA, Connolly LE, Deavers MT, Malpica A, McCluggage WG. High-grade ovarian serous carcinoma exhibits significantly higher p16 expression than low-grade serous carcinoma and serous borderline tumour. Histopathology. 2007;50:773–9.
12. Vang R, Shih Ie M, Kurman RJ. Ovarian low-grade and high-grade serous carcinoma: pathogenesis, clinicopathologic and molecular biologic features, and diagnostic problems. Adv Anat Pathol. 2009;16:267–82.

13. Zivanovic O, Sima CS, Iasonos A, Bell-McGuinn KM, Sabbatini PJ, Leitao MM, Levine DA, Gardner GJ, Barakat RR, Chi DS. Exploratory analysis of serum CA-125 response to surgery and the risk of relapse in patients with FIGO stage IIIC ovarian cancer. Gynecol Oncol. 2009;115:209–14.
14. Seidman JD, Horkayne-Szakaly I, Cosin JA, Ryu HS, Haiba M, Boice CR, Yemelyanova AV. Testing of two binary grading systems for FIGO stage III serous carcinoma of the ovary and peritoneum. Gynecol Oncol. 2006;103:703–8.
15. Motohara T, Tashiro H, Miyahara Y, Sakaguchi I, Ohtake H, Katabuchi H. Long-term oncological outcomes of ovarian serous carcinomas with psammoma bodies: a novel insight into the molecular pathogenesis of ovarian epithelial carcinoma. Cancer Sci. 2010;101:1550–6.
16. Hannibal CG, Vang R, Junge J, Kjaerbye-Thygesen A, Kurman RJ, Kjaer SK. A binary histologic grading system for ovarian serous carcinoma is an independent prognostic factor: a population-based study of 4317 women diagnosed in Denmark 1978-2006. Gynecol Oncol. 2012;125:655–60.
17. Eisenkop SM, Spirtos NM, Lin WC. "Optimal" cytoreduction for advanced epithelial ovarian cancer: a commentary. Gynecol Oncol. 2006;103:329–35.
18. Zhang S, Royer R, Li S, McLaughlin JR, Rosen B, Risch HA, Fan I, Bradley L, Shaw PA, Narod SA. Frequencies of BRCA1 and BRCA2 mutations among 1,342 unselected patients with invasive ovarian cancer. Gynecol Oncol. 2011;121:353–7.
19. Cancer Genome Atlas Research Network. Integrated genomic analyses of ovarian carcinoma. Nature. 2011;474:609–15.
20. Verhaak RG, Tamayo P, Yang JY, Hubbard D, Zhang H, Creighton CJ, Fereday S, Lawrence M, Carter SL, Mermel CH, Kostic AD, Etemadmoghadam D, Saksena G, Cibulskis K, Duraisamy S, Levanon K, Sougnez C, Tsherniak A, Gomez S, Onofrio R, Gabriel S, Chin L, Zhang N, Spellman PT, Zhang Y, Akbani R, Hoadley KA, Kahn A, Kobel M, Huntsman D, Soslow RA, Defazio A, Birrer MJ, Gray JW, Weinstein JN, Bowtell DD, Drapkin R, Mesirov JP, Getz G, Levine DA, Meyerson M. Prognostically relevant gene signatures of high-grade serous ovarian carcinoma. J Clin Invest. 2013;123:517–25.
21. Murakami R, Matsumura N, Mandai M, Yoshihara K, Tanabe H, Nakai H, Yamanoi K, Abiko K, Yoshioka Y, Hamanishi J, Yamaguchi K, Baba T, Koshiyama M, Enomoto T, Okamoto A, Murphy SK, Mori S, Mikami Y, Minamiguchi S, Konishi I. Establishment of a novel histopathological classification of high-grade serous ovarian carcinoma correlated with prognostically distinct gene expression subtypes. Am J Pathol. 2016;186:1103–13.
22. Auersperg N, Wong AS, Choi KC, Kang SK, Leung PC. Ovarian surface epithelium: biology, endocrinology, and pathology. Endocr Rev. 2001;22:255–88.
23. Piek JM, van Diest PJ, Zweemer RP, Jansen JW, Poort-Keesom RJ, Menko FH, Gille JJ, Jongsma AP, Pals G, Kenemans P, Verheijen RH. Dysplastic changes in prophylactically removed fallopian tubes of women predisposed to developing ovarian cancer. J Pathol. 2001;195:451–6.
24. Medeiros F, Muto MG, Lee Y, Elvin JA, Callahan MJ, Feltmate C, Garber JE, Cramer DW, Crum CP. The tubal fimbria is a preferred site for early adenocarcinoma in women with familial ovarian cancer syndrome. Am J Surg Pathol. 2006;30:230–6.
25. Kindelberger DW, Lee Y, Miron A, Hirsch MS, Feltmate C, Medeiros F, Callahan MJ, Garner EO, Gordon RW, Birch C, Berkowitz RS, Muto MG, Crum CP. Intraepithelial carcinoma of the fimbria and pelvic serous carcinoma: evidence for a causal relationship. Am J Surg Pathol. 2007;31:161–9.
26. Colgan TJ, Murphy J, Cole DE, Narod S, Rosen B. Occult carcinoma in prophylactic oophorectomy specimens: prevalence and association with BRCA germline mutation status. Am J Surg Pathol. 2001;25:1283–9.
27. Callahan MJ, Crum CP, Medeiros F, Kindelberger DW, Elvin JA, Garber JE, Feltmate CM, Berkowitz RS, Muto MG. Primary fallopian tube malignancies in BRCA-positive women undergoing surgery for ovarian cancer risk reduction. J Clin Oncol. 2007;25:3985–90.
28. Finch A, Shaw P, Rosen B, Murphy J, Narod SA, Colgan TJ. Clinical and pathologic findings of prophylactic salpingo-oophorectomies in 159 BRCA1 and BRCA2 carriers. Gynecol Oncol. 2006;100:58–64.
29. Roh MH, Kindelberger D, Crum CP. Serous tubal intraepithelial carcinoma and the dominant ovarian mass: clues to serous tumor origin? Am J Surg Pathol. 2009;33:376–83.
30. Tang S, Onuma K, Deb P, Wang E, Lytwyn A, Sur M, Daya D. Frequency of serous tubal intraepithelial carcinoma in various gynecologic malignancies: a study of 300 consecutive cases. Int J Gynecol Pathol. 2012;31:103–10.
31. Przybycin CG, Kurman RJ, Ronnett BM, Shih Ie M, Vang R. Are all pelvic (nonuterine) serous carcinomas of tubal origin? Am J Surg Pathol. 2010;34:1407–16.
32. Gilks CB, Irving J, Kobel M, Lee C, Singh N, Wilkinson N, McCluggage WG. Incidental nonuterine high-grade serous carcinomas arise in the fallopian tube in most cases: further evidence for the tubal origin of high-grade serous carcinomas. Am J Surg Pathol. 2015;39:357–64.
33. Carlson JW, Miron A, Jarboe EA, Parast MM, Hirsch MS, Lee Y, Muto MG, Kindelberger D, Crum CP. Serous tubal intraepithelial carcinoma: its potential role in primary peritoneal serous carcinoma and serous cancer prevention. J Clin Oncol. 2008;26:4160–5.
34. Salvador S, Rempel A, Soslow RA, Gilks B, Huntsman D, Miller D. Chromosomal instability in fallopian tube precursor lesions of serous carcinoma and frequent monoclonality of synchronous ovarian and fallopian tube mucosal serous carcinoma. Gynecol Oncol. 2008;110:408–17.
35. Kuhn E, Meeker A, Wang TL, Sehdev AS, Kurman RJ, Shih Ie M. Shortened telomeres in serous tubal intraepithelial carcinoma: an early event in ovarian high-grade serous carcinogenesis. Am J Surg Pathol. 2010;34:829–36.
36. Kuhn E, Wang TL, Doberstein K, Bahadirli-Talbott A, Ayhan A, Sehdev AS, Drapkin R, Kurman RJ, Shih Ie M. CCNE1 amplification and centrosome number abnormality in serous tubal intraepithelial carcinoma: further evidence supporting its role as a precursor of ovarian high-grade serous carcinoma. Mod Pathol. 2016;29:1254–61.
37. Singh N, Gilks CB, Wilkinson N, McCluggage WG. Assessment of a new system for primary site assignment in high-grade serous carcinoma of the fallopian tube, ovary, and peritoneum. Histopathology. 2015;67:331–7.
38. Prat J. Abridged republication of FIGO's staging classification for cancer of the ovary, fallopian tube, and peritoneum. Cancer. 2015;121(19):3452–4.
39. Singh N, Gilks CB, Wilkinson N, McCluggage WG. Assignment of primary site in high-grade serous tubal, ovarian and peritoneal carcinoma: a proposal. Histopathology. 2014;65:149–54.
40. McCluggage WG, Judge MJ, Clarke BA, Davidson B, Gilks CB, Hollema H, Ledermann JA, Matias-Guiu X, Mikami Y, Stewart CJ, Vang R, Hirschowitz L. Data set for reporting of ovary, fallopian tube and primary peritoneal carcinoma: recommendations from the International Collaboration on Cancer Reporting (ICCR). Mod Pathol. 2015;28:1101–22.
41. Prat J. Ovarian, fallopian tube and peritoneal cancer staging: rationale and explanation of new FIGO staging 2013. Best Pract Res Clin Obstet Gynaecol. 2015;29:858–69.
42. Gilks CB, Miller D. Opportunistic salpingectomy for women at low risk for development of ovarian carcinoma: the time has come. Gynecol Oncol. 2013;129:443–4.
43. McAlpine JN, Tone AA, Hanley GE. Opportunistic salpingectomy: we chose to act, not wait. J Obstet Gynaecol. 2016;38:425–7.
44. Kho RM, Wechter ME. Operative outcomes of opportunistic bilateral salpingectomy at the time of benign hysterectomy in low-risk premenopausal women: a systematic review. J Minim Invasive Gynecol. 2017;24:218–29.
45. Hanley GE, McAlpine JN, Kwon JS, Mitchell G. Opportunistic salpingectomy for ovarian cancer prevention. Gynecol Oncol Res Pract. 2015;2:5.

46. Meserve EE, Brouwer J, Crum CP. Serous tubal intraepithelial neoplasia: the concept and its application. Mod Pathol. 2017;30:710.
47. Nafisi H, Ghorab Z, Ismill N, Dube V, Plotkin A, Han G, Cesari M, Lu FI, Saad R, Khalifa M, Nofech-Mozes S. Immunophenotypic analysis in early Mullerian serous carcinogenesis. Int J Gynecol Pathol. 2015;34:424–36.
48. Visvanathan K, Vang R, Shaw P, Gross A, Soslow R, Parkash V, Shih Ie M, Kurman RJ. Diagnosis of serous tubal intraepithelial carcinoma based on morphologic and immunohistochemical features: a reproducibility study. Am J Surg Pathol. 2011;35:1766–75.
49. Vang R, Visvanathan K, Gross A, Maambo E, Gupta M, Kuhn E, Li RF, Ronnett BM, Seidman JD, Yemelyanova A, Shih Ie M, Shaw PA, Soslow RA, Kurman RJ. Validation of an algorithm for the diagnosis of serous tubal intraepithelial carcinoma. Int J Gynecol Pathol. 2012;31:243–53.
50. Kobel M, Kalloger SE, Carrick J, Huntsman D, Asad H, Oliva E, Ewanowich CA, Soslow RA, Gilks CB. A limited panel of immunomarkers can reliably distinguish between clear cell and high-grade serous carcinoma of the ovary. Am J Surg Pathol. 2009;33:14–21.
51. Jarboe E, Folkins A, Nucci MR, Kindelberger D, Drapkin R, Miron A, Lee Y, Crum CP. Serous carcinogenesis in the fallopian tube: a descriptive classification. Int J Gynecol Pathol. 2008;27:1–9.
52. Jarboe EA, Miron A, Carlson JW, Hirsch MS, Kindelberger D, Mutter GL, Crum CP, Nucci MR. Coexisting intraepithelial serous carcinomas of the endometrium and fallopian tube: frequency and potential significance. Int J Gynecol Pathol. 2009;28:308–15.
53. Rabban JT, Vohra P, Zaloudek CJ. Nongynecologic metastases to fallopian tube mucosa: a potential mimic of tubal high-grade serous carcinoma and benign tubal mucinous metaplasia or nonmucinous hyperplasia. Am J Surg Pathol. 2015;39:35–51.
54. Stewart CJ, Leung YC, Whitehouse A. Fallopian tube metastases of non-gynaecological origin: a series of 20 cases emphasizing patterns of involvement including intra-epithelial spread. Histopathology. 2012;60:E106–14.
55. Folkins AK, Jarboe EA, Saleemuddin A, Lee Y, Callahan MJ, Drapkin R, Garber JE, Muto MG, Tworoger S, Crum CP. A candidate precursor to pelvic serous cancer (p53 signature) and its prevalence in ovaries and fallopian tubes from women with BRCA mutations. Gynecol Oncol. 2008;109:168–73.
56. Mingels MJ, Roelofsen T, van der Laak JA, de Hullu JA, van Ham MA, Massuger LF, Bulten J, Bol M. Tubal epithelial lesions in salpingo-oophorectomy specimens of BRCA-mutation carriers and controls. Gynecol Oncol. 2012;127:88–93.
57. Poon C, Hyde S, Grant P, Newman M, Ireland Jenkin K. Incidence and characteristics of unsuspected neoplasia discovered in high-risk women undergoing risk reductive bilateral Salpingooophorectomy. Int J Gynecol Cancer. 2016;26:1415–20.
58. Powell CB, Kenley E, Chen LM, Crawford B, McLennan J, Zaloudek C, Komaromy M, Beattie M, Ziegler J. Risk-reducing salpingo-oophorectomy in BRCA mutation carriers: role of serial sectioning in the detection of occult malignancy. J Clin Oncol. 2005;23:127–32.
59. Rabban JT, Garg K, Crawford B, Chen LM, Zaloudek CJ. Early detection of high-grade tubal serous carcinoma in women at low risk for hereditary breast and ovarian cancer syndrome by systematic examination of fallopian tubes incidentally removed during benign surgery. Am J Surg Pathol. 2014;38:729–42.
60. Brown PO, Palmer C. The preclinical natural history of serous ovarian cancer: defining the target for early detection. PLoS Med. 2009;6:e1000114.
61. Bell DA. Low-grade serous tumors of ovary. Int J Gynecol Pathol. 2014;33:348–56.
62. Bodurka DC, Deavers MT, Tian C, Sun CC, Malpica A, Coleman RL, Lu KH, Sood AK, Birrer MJ, Ozols R, Baergen R, Emerson RE, Steinhoff M, Behmaram B, Rasty G, Gershenson DM. Reclassification of serous ovarian carcinoma by a 2-tier system: a Gynecologic Oncology Group Study. Cancer. 2012;118: 3087–94.
63. Hannibal CG, Vang R, Junge J, Frederiksen K, Kurman RJ, Kjaer SK. A nationwide study of ovarian serous borderline tumors in Denmark 1978-2002. Risk of recurrence, and development of ovarian serous carcinoma. Gynecol Oncol. 2017;144:174–80.
64. Gershenson DM, Sun CC, Lu KH, Coleman RL, Sood AK, Malpica A, Deavers MT, Silva EG, Bodurka DC. Clinical behavior of stage II-IV low-grade serous carcinoma of the ovary. Obstet Gynecol. 2006;108:361–8.
65. Cho KR, Shih Ie M. Ovarian cancer. Annu Rev Pathol. 2009;4:287–313.
66. Farley J, Brady WE, Vathipadiekal V, Lankes HA, Coleman R, Morgan MA, Mannel R, Yamada SD, Mutch D, Rodgers WH, Birrer M, Gershenson DM. Selumetinib in women with recurrent low-grade serous carcinoma of the ovary or peritoneum: an open-label, single-arm, phase 2 study. Lancet Oncol. 2013;14:134–40.
67. Ho CL, Kurman RJ, Dehari R, Wang TL, Shih Ie M. Mutations of BRAF and KRAS precede the development of ovarian serous borderline tumors. Cancer Res. 2004;64:6915–8.
68. Maniar KP, Wang Y, Visvanathan K, Shih Ie M, Kurman RJ. Evaluation of microinvasion and lymph node involvement in ovarian serous borderline/atypical proliferative serous tumors: a morphologic and immunohistochemical analysis of 37 cases. Am J Surg Pathol. 2014;38:743–55.
69. Barcena C, Oliva E. WT1 expression in the female genital tract. Adv Anat Pathol. 2011;18:454–65.
70. Escobar J, Klimowicz AC, Dean M, Chu P, Nation JG, Nelson GS, Ghatage P, Kalloger SE, Kobel M. Quantification of ER/PR expression in ovarian low-grade serous carcinoma. Gynecol Oncol. 2013;128:371–6.
71. Laury AR, Hornick JL, Perets R, Krane JF, Corson J, Drapkin R, Hirsch MS. PAX8 reliably distinguishes ovarian serous tumors from malignant mesothelioma. Am J Surg Pathol. 2010;34:627–35.
72. Bell KA, Smith Sehdev AE, Kurman RJ. Refined diagnostic criteria for implants associated with ovarian atypical proliferative serous tumors (borderline) and micropapillary serous carcinomas. Am J Surg Pathol. 2001;25:419–32.
73. Hauptmann S, Friedrich K, Redline R, Avril S. Ovarian borderline tumors in the 2014 WHO classification: evolving concepts and diagnostic criteria. Virchows Arch. 2017;470:125–42.
74. Deavers MT, Gershenson DM, Tortolero-Luna G, Malpica A, Lu KH, Silva EG. Micropapillary and cribriform patterns in ovarian serous tumors of low malignant potential: a study of 99 advanced stage cases. Am J Surg Pathol. 2002;26:1129–41.
75. Gotlieb WH, Chetrit A, Menczer J, Hirsh-Yechezkel G, Lubin F, Friedman E, Modan B, Ben-Baruch G. Demographic and genetic characteristics of patients with borderline ovarian tumors as compared to early stage invasive ovarian cancer. Gynecol Oncol. 2005;97:780–3.
76. Seidman JD, Kurman RJ. Ovarian serous borderline tumors: a critical review of the literature with emphasis on prognostic indicators. Hum Pathol. 2000;31:539–57.
77. Burks RT, Sherman ME, Kurman RJ. Micropapillary serous carcinoma of the ovary. A distinctive low-grade carcinoma related to serous borderline tumors. Am J Surg Pathol. 1996;20:1319–30.
78. Smith Sehdev AE, Sehdev PS, Kurman RJ. Noninvasive and invasive micropapillary (low-grade) serous carcinoma of the ovary: a clinicopathologic analysis of 135 cases. Am J Surg Pathol. 2003;27:725–36.
79. Gershenson DM, Silva EG, Levy L, Burke TW, Wolf JK, Tornos C. Ovarian serous borderline tumors with invasive peritoneal implants. Cancer. 1998;82:1096–103.

Ovarian Carcinoma Associated with Endometriosis

5

Masanori Yasuda and Mitsutake Yano

Abstract

Endometrioid carcinoma (EMC) and clear cell carcinoma (CCC) are the representatives of endometriosis-associated ovarian tumor. In addition, seromucinous tumors (so far designated as mixed müllerian tumor), mainly composed of borderline tumor, are also associated with endometriosis in their tumorigenesis. In many of these tumors, endometriosis is regarded as a precursor. Therefore, EMCs, CCCs, and seromucinous tumors as well as other epithelial tumors may not be originated from the ovary, in which a soil permissive for these cancers is proposed to be provided.

Endometriosis (endometrioma) is nowadays interpreted as benign endometrioid tumor according to the revised WHO classification. For EMC, atypical endometriosis may play a role in its evolution, while endometrioid borderline tumor has little association with the development of EMC. When given the low-grade ovarian EMC and endometrial EMC at the same time, they may be independent to a large extent because of good prognosis of the patient. The adenocarcinofibroma type of CCC is often found to have a transition with benign and borderline counterparts, showing a continuous range of tumorigenetic spectrum from benign to malignant.

EMC is divided into low-grade as type I and high-grade as type II. CCC also can be categorized into type I tumors. Certain genetic abnormalities, such as phosphatase and tensin homolog deleted from chromosome 10 (*PTEN*), AT-rich interactive domain 1A (*ARID1A*), *and PIK3CA,* are often shared by endometriosis/endometriotic cyst (endometrioma), EMCs, CCCs, and seromucinous tumors. But, the cellular origin of these tumors remains to be characterized.

Keywords

Endometriosis · Endometrioid carcinoma · Clear cell carcinoma · Seromucinous tumor

5.1 General (Fig. 5.1)

Following serous carcinoma (SEC), endometrioid carcinoma (EMC) is the second most common ovarian carcinoma and prevalent in the fifth and sixth decades, accounting for 10–15% of the ovarian carcinomas [1]. However, when strict criteria are used (i.e., some of high-grade EMCs are reclassified as high-grade SEC), the frequency of EMC may fall to <10% [2]. The third most common is clear cell carcinoma (CCC) worldwide, although in Japan CCC accounts for a higher proportion relative to western countries [3–5], nearly reaching the frequency of SEC [6, 7]. The mean patient age is 56 [8] or 58 [9] years old for EMC and 55 years old for CCC [3]. Thirty-one percent of EMCs are stage I (vs. 43% for stage I [10]), 20% are stage II, 38% are stage III, and 11% are stage IV [11]. In CCCs, 35–60% are stage I, 10–22% are stage II, 29% are stage III, and 9% are stage IV [11]. In Japan, stage IC cases are the most prevalent [12].

The association with ipsilateral ovarian or pelvic endometriosis is noted in up to 42% of EMCs [13–15] and 50–70% of CCCs [16, 17], respectively. The presence of endometriosis increases the risk of CCC and EMC by up to 3 times [18, 19]. There is a frequent coexistence of the ovarian EMC with endometrial EMC [20–22]. The age of patients whose ovarian EMC is associated with endometriosis is 5–10 years lower than that of EMC without associated endometriosis [9]. The 5-year survival ratio of patients with stage I EMC is 78%; stage II, 63%; stage III, 24%; and stage IV, 6% [1]. Patients with grade 3 EMC have a more unfavorable prognosis than those with grade 1 or 2 EMC. The 5-year survival ratio of patients with stage I CCC is 88%; stage II, 70%; stage III, 33%; and stage IV, 0% [23].

M. Yasuda (✉) · M. Yano
Department of Pathology, Saitama Medical University International Medical Center,
Hidaka City, Saitama Prefecture, Japan
e-mail: m_yasuda@saitama-med.ac.jp

T. Moriya (ed.), *Pathology of Female Cancers*, https://doi.org/10.1007/978-981-10-8606-9_5

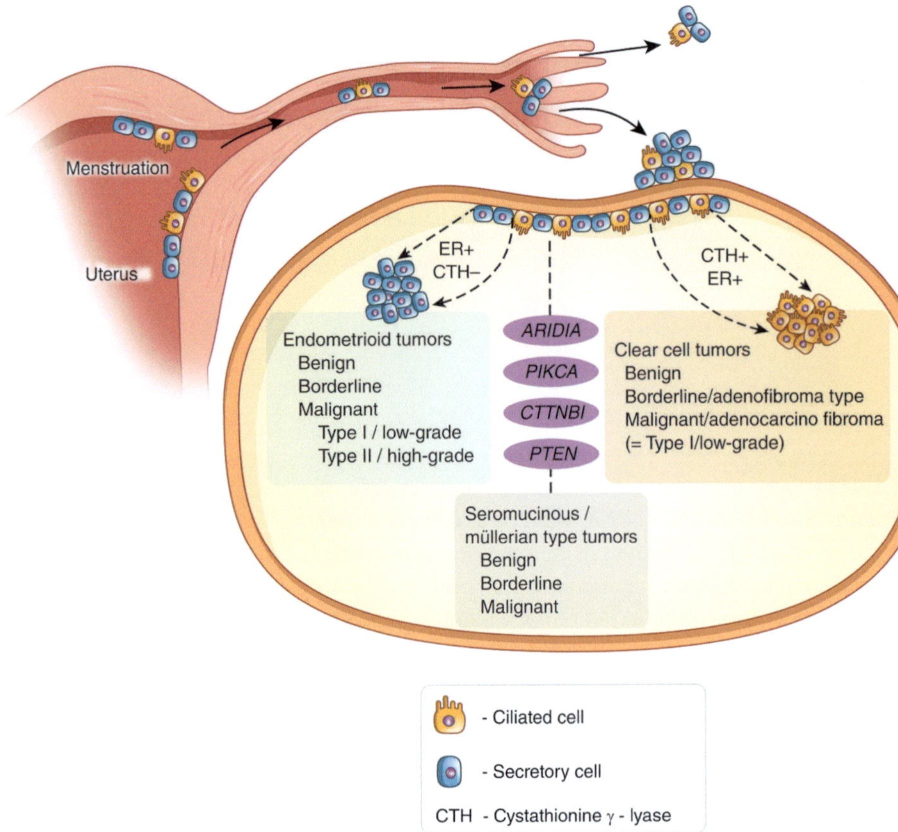

Fig. 5.1 Tumorigenesis/development of endometriosis-associated ovarian tumors

Seromucinous tumors, or the so-called müllerian mixed tumors, have been newly added in ovarian epithelial tumors in the WHO classification 2014 and are composed of benign, borderline, and malignant subtypes. Seromucinous borderline tumor/atypical proliferative seromucinous tumor, representing seromucinous tumors, has been designated as endocervical-like mucinous borderline tumor and often occurs bilaterally, showing a close association with endometriosis in tumorigenesis. Seromucinous carcinoma is a rare ovarian tumor for which, so far, the clinicopathological independency as a disease entity has to be established [24].

According to the recently proposed dualistic model of carcinogenesis which divided epithelial ovarian cancers into two broad categories, low-grade EMC and CCC comprise type I tumors [25]. On the other hand, high-grade EMC is included in type II tumors. Type I tumors are generally indolent and present as stage I and are characterized by specific mutations, which differ from those seen in type II tumors. Type I and type II tumors develop independently along different genetic pathways [25].

The precise origin of endometriosis has not been completely established, but the preponderance of date favors whether endometriosis develops from retrograde menstrual flow [25, 26]. The epidemiologic evidence that a protective effect by tubal ligation is seen only for EMC and CCC supports the hypothesis that both carcinomas arise in endometrial tissues implanted on the ovary [25, 27]. Therefore, many of the EMCs, CCCs, and seromucinous tumors may not be called the ovarian-origin tumors.

5.2 Endometriosis/Endometriotic Cyst (Fig. 5.2)

Ectopic presence of endometrial glands and stromal cells is designated as endometriosis, which affects approximately 10% of reproductive-age women and as high as 35–50% of women with infertility [28]. Endometriosis is considered mostly to originate from endometrial tissues, which implant on the ovary and peritoneal surface after retrograde flow of menstruation from uterine cavity via the fallopian tube [29]. This theory is supported by the evidence that increased risk of endometriosis is related to an increased exposure to menstruation, i.e., longer duration of flow or high volumes of retrograde menstruation in states where estrogenic stimulation is maintained [30, 31]. The risk of endometriosis can be reduced by the usage of contraceptive medication, but intrauterine device or diaphragm does not have the effect on the risk reduction [32]. Endometriotic lesions are characterized by cancer-like features such as local invasion and resistance to apoptosis [33]. It was found that endometriotic lesions in deep infiltrating endometriosis, which are associated with no risk of malig-

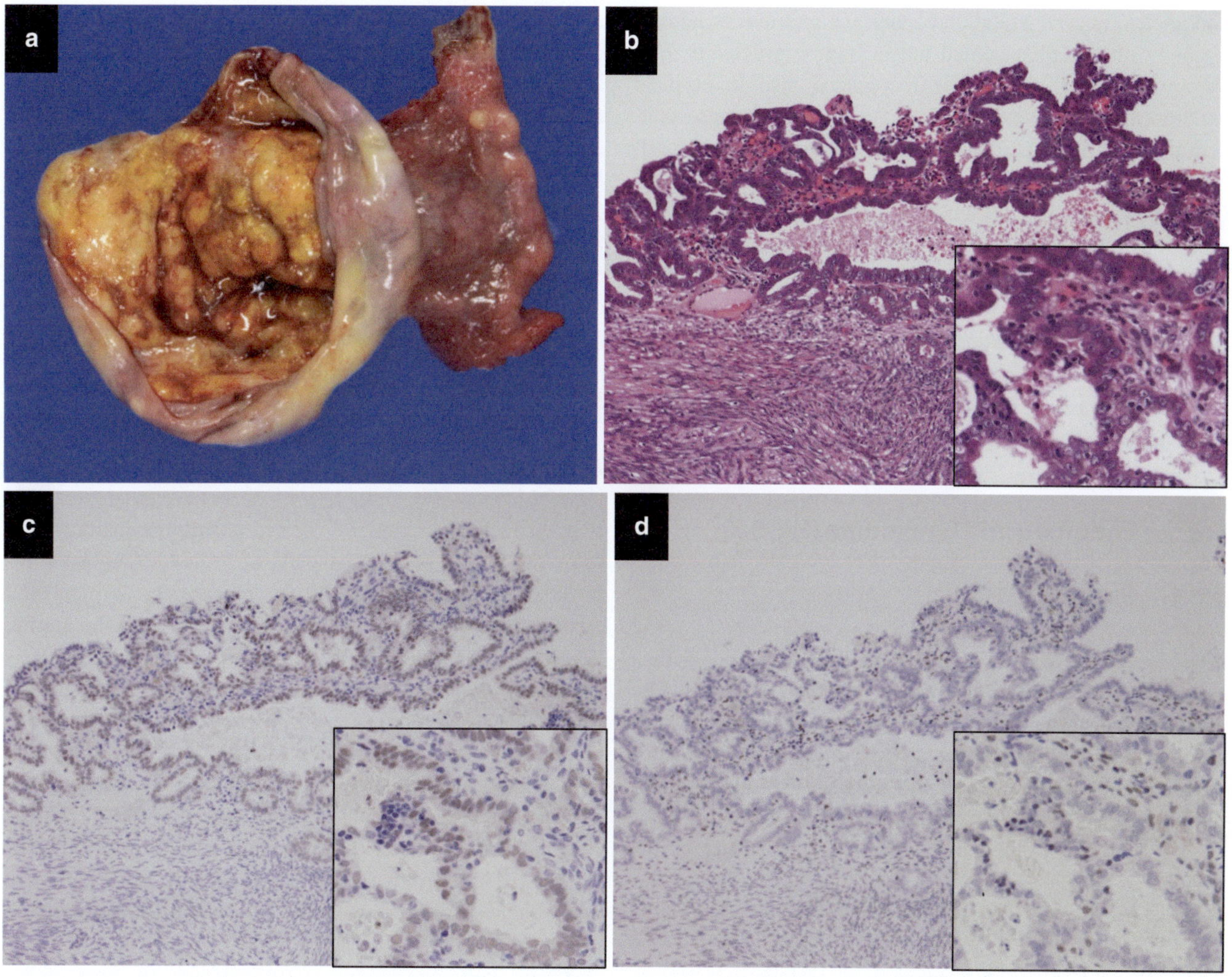

Fig. 5.2 Atypical endometriosis. (**a**) In the cystic lesion of the ovary, low-elevated nodular or papillary parts are observed. (**b**) On the inner surface, variable-sized glands are observed to be aggregated, mimicking atypical endometrial hyperplasia (H&E, inset: high-powered view). (**c**) The glandular cells show a positive reaction for HNF1β, but the stromal cells are negative (immunohistochemistry, inset: high-powered view). (**d**) No positive reaction of ARID1A is observed in the glandular cells, but the stromal cells are positive (immunohistochemistry, inset: high-powered view)

nant transformation, harbor somatic cancer driver mutations in AT-rich interactive domain 1A (*ARID1A*), phosphatdylinositol 3-kinase (*PIK3CA*), *KRAS, or PPP2R1A* [33].

In the WHO classification 2003, benign endometrioid tumors were subclassified into cystadenoma, adenofibroma, and cystadenofibroma. However, there have been no convincing epidemiological data with these tumors because of the rarity. Endometriotic cyst, the cystic form of endometriosis (endometrioma), has been defined as benign endometrioid tumor in the WHO classification 2014 for the first time and is usually complicated with endometriosis elsewhere.

Basically, endometriosis is composed of endometrial glands which are surrounded by endometrial stroma. The glandular cells are usually tall and columnar with elongate cigar-like nuclei showing regular vertical orientation [29]. There are variable metaplastic changes designated as mucinous, serous/tubal, ciliated, secretory, clear cell, and squamous. In the differential diagnoses of endometrioid tumors, a lack of endometrial stroma, i.e., presence of abundant dense fibrotic stroma, is supportive of endometrioid cystadenoma/adenofibroma. Endometriotic cyst (endometrioma) typically has dark brown hemorrhagic contents, therefore being designated as chocolate cyst as a clinical term. In the cases with little or no lining cells and ambiguous association of stromal cells in the cystic lesions, hemosiderin-laden macrophages and fibrosis become the indicators of endometriotic cyst. In the older lesions, xanthomatous changes may be prominent [1]. However, endometrioid cystadenoma/adenofibroma may develop within the endometriotic cyst.

The development of endometrioid, clear cell, and seromucinous tumors is histopathologically and genetically implicated to have been closely associated with endometriosis/

endometriotic cyst. Mutation of *ARID1A* and loss of heterozygosity of phosphatase and tensin homolog deleted from chromosome 10 (*PTEN*) are recognized also in atypical endometrial cells of endometriosis (Fig. 5.2), which are adjacent to EMC and CCC. Some mutations and genomic landscape features are more likely to be found in one of EMC and CCC; however, it is not able to identify a single class of mutations that was exclusively present in one of these histologic types and not the other [18]. Using a proteomic screen, CCC may be derived from ciliated cell lineage of endometrial cells of eutopic endometrium and endometriosis, with the specific expression of cystathionine gamma-lyase (CTH) [18]. In contrast, EMC may be derived from the secretory cell lineage.

5.3 Endometrioid Carcinoma (Fig. 5.3)

5.3.1 Gross

EMC develops basically as a solid and soft mass with a smooth surface, measuring a mean size of 15 cm [1]. The cystic space is often complicated with a solid part and partly contains papillae. In the case of EMC associated with endometriotic cyst, it tends to be a polypoid lesion protruding into the lumen of thick-walled cyst, filled with bloody contents.

5.3.2 Histopathology (Fig. 5.3)

The cells of EMC, which are defined as having a resemblance to endometrial EMC, are arranged in tubular and papillary nests with back-to-back, confluent, or cribriform patterns. A destructive or infiltrative manner with desmoplastic reaction is less frequently exhibited. The ovarian EMC is categorized into three grades according to the grading scheme applied in the endometrial EMC, primarily based on the architecture: with those having 5% or less of solid growth considered grade 1; those with between 6 and 50% solid growth considered grade 2; and those with more than 50% solid growth considered grade 3 [34]. Most EMCs are well differentiated, classified as grade 1 or 2 (i.e., low-grade EMC). Poorly differentiated EMCs, i.e., grade 3 EMC (i.e., high-grade EMC), are composed of a predominantly solid part with focal abortive glandular areas. The presence of grade 3 nuclei involving more than 50% of the tumor is associated with more aggressive behavior, therefore being justified upgrading the tumor by one grade [22].

Several variants are seen in endometrial EMC: squamous differentiation, mostly taking the form of morule; secretory changes; rare settings of mucin-rich, ciliated cells, oxyphilic and spindle cell types; and mimics of sex cord-stromal tumors such as Sertoli cell tumor or adult-type granulosa cell tumor. Squamous differentiation, found in 30–50% [35], does not warrant upgrading [36], since it usually fails to affect the prognosis adversely. Peritoneal foreign body granulomas with phagocytosis of keratinized substances, which may be found in EMC with squamous differentiation, have little prognostic significance when the granuloma does not contain viable carcinoma cells. Functioning stroma, which typically produces sex steroid hormones represented by estrogen (mainly estradiol), is recognizable in EMC, especially in a variant resembling sex cord-stromal tumor.

5.3.3 Differential Diagnoses

Borderline endometrioid tumor/atypical proliferative endometrioid tumor (Fig. 5.4): These tumors have two representative growth patterns of being adenofibromatous and intracystic. The proliferative cells with crowded and back-to-back arrangement are mildly to moderately atypical and analogous to atypical endometrial hyperplasia of the uterine body. Also commonly observed is squamous/morular differentiation, which should not be mistaken for stromal invasion.

Serous carcinoma (SEC): Distinguishing high-grade EMC from high-grade SEC may be difficult because they may share the same immunohistochemical profile. Glandular pattern and squamous differentiation can be the indicator suggestive of high-grade EMC, while papillary arrangement and solid nest structure with slit-like narrow spaces favor the diagnosis of high-grade SEC.

Clear cell carcinoma (CCC): Refer to Sect. 5.4.3 (Figs. 5.5 and 5.6).

Sex cord-stromal tumor: EMC occasionally resembles sex cord-stromal tumors such as Sertoli cell tumor and adult-type granulosa cell tumor. In the EMC with Sertoli cell tumor pattern, there are hollow or solid tubules. On the other hand, solid nests with punctuation and rosette-like structure, simulating microglandular/follicular pattern, are indicative of adult-type granulosa cell tumor. Functioning stroma with serum elevation of estrogen (e.g., estradiol) is also often encountered in EMC resembling sex cord-stromal tumor [37].

5.3.4 Immunohistochemistry

Pax-8: Most EMCs express Pax-8, which is a member of the paired box (*PAX*) family of transcription factor gene and is usually helpful in distinguishing müllerian tract origin tumors from malignant mesothelioma and some metastatic carcinomas of breast, colon and lung origin. Pax-8 is strongly expressed in 75% of EMCs [38] but is also highly sensitive for thyroid, renal, and thymic tumors.

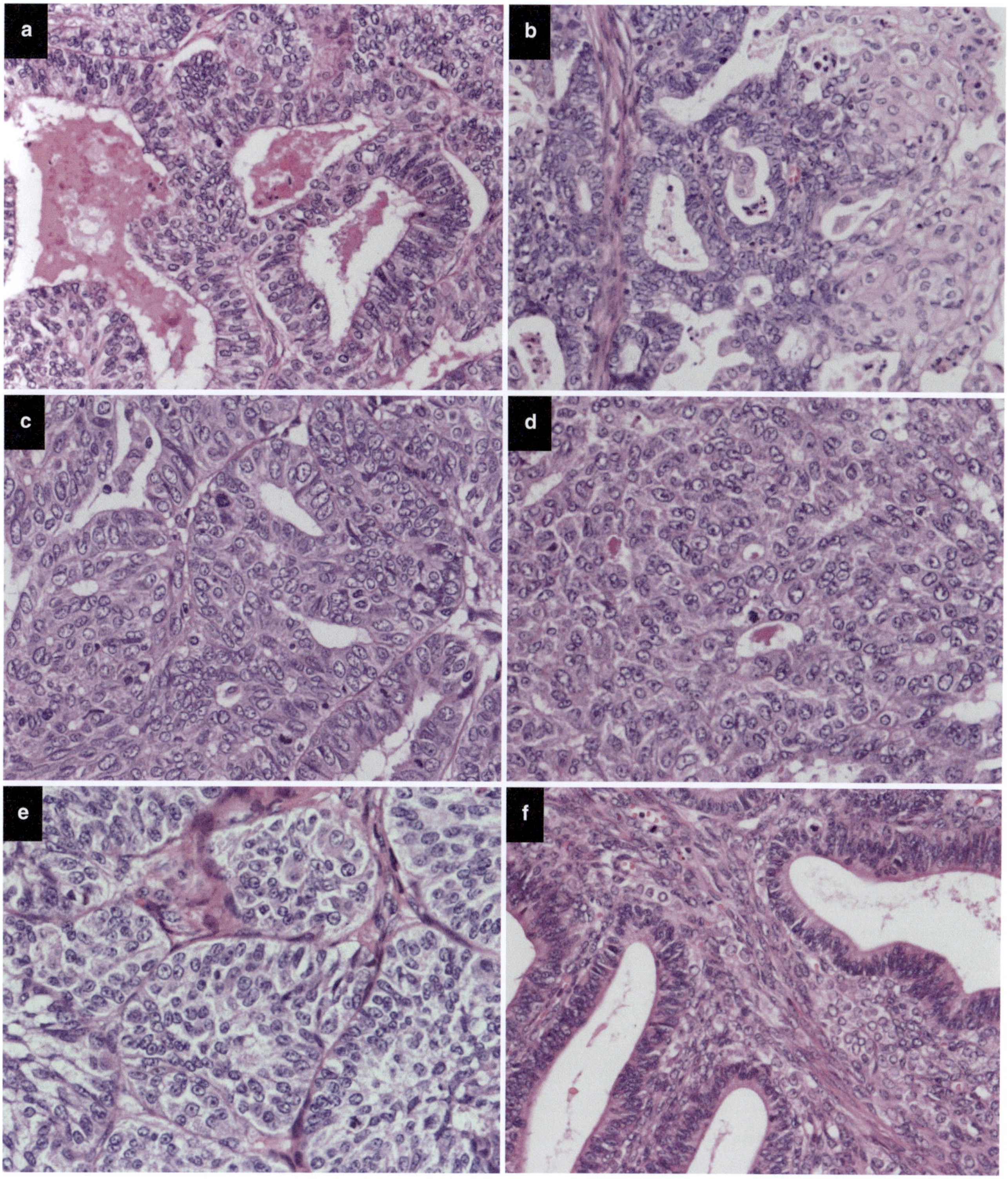

Fig. 5.3 Endometrioid carcinoma (EMC). (**a**) The atypical columnar cells are arranged in a well-formed tubular manner but focally fused, diagnosed as G1 EMC (H&E). (**b**) The tumor cells of G1 EMC show squamous differentiation (H&E). (**c**) There is a transition between glandular and solid components instead of morular forms, diagnosed as G2 EMC (H&E). (**d**) Solid components are more predominant with focally vague glandular structure, diagnosed as G3 EMC (H&E). (**e**) The tumor cells are forming solid nests looking like adult-type granular cell tumor, diagnosed as EMC characteristic of a resemblance to sex cord-stromal tumor (H&E). (**f**) The tumor has an abundant functioning stroma intervening between glands of G1 EMC, composed of cells with thecoma-like features and those with luteinization (H&E)

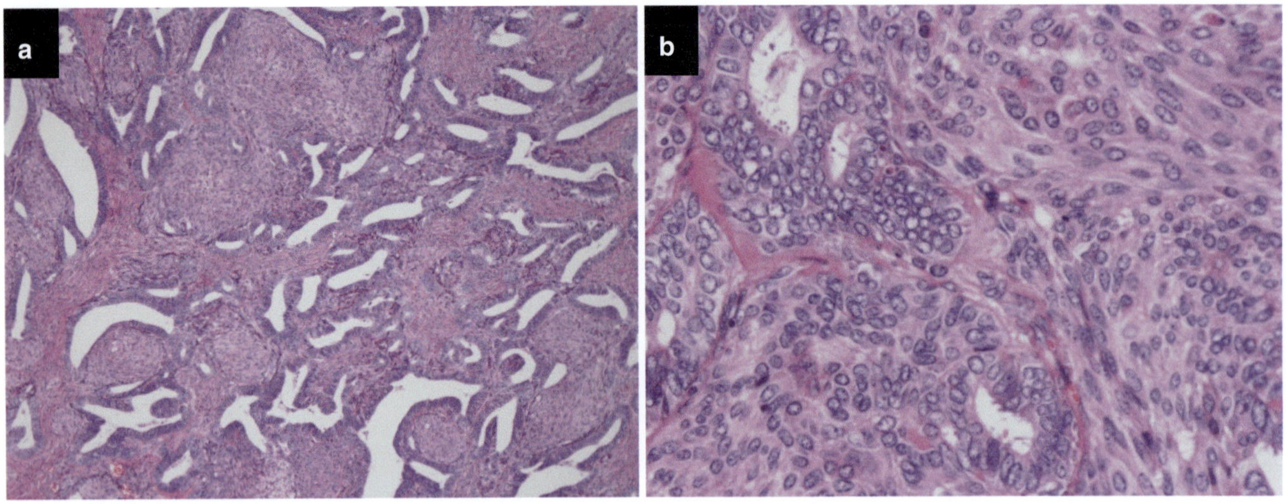

Fig. 5.4 Endometrioid borderline tumor. (**a**) Glandular and solid components are admixed with a relative predominance of solid components (H&E). (**b**) Mildly atypical columnar cells are transitioning with morular cells (solid components), reminiscent of atypical endometrial hyperplasia (H&E)

Vimentin: Approximately 33% of EMC show basal membranous and/or cytoplasmic staining [39].

β-Catenin: Compared to other ovarian carcinomas, EMC is most likely to show the nuclear and cytoplasmic positive reaction [40], showing that a majority of them have *CTNNB1* mutation. β-Catenin expression is associated with low-grade, low-stage, morular, or squamous differentiation and also favorable prognosis. β-Catenin and CDX-2 are expressed in the nuclei of morulae, and CD10 shows cytoplasmic staining [41, 42].

Markers for differentiation from sex cord-stromal tumors: EMC is positive for epithelial membrane antigen (EMA), but does not positively react with inhibin-α and calretinin [43, 44]. Sex cord-stromal tumor may stain for cytokeratin, but may be negative for EMA, and shows cytoplasmic reaction for inhibin-α and nuclear reaction for calretinin. FOX-L2 is sensitive and specific for adult-type granulosa cell tumor.

Markers for differentiation from metastatic carcinoma: Many metastatic colorectal carcinomas mimic EMC. CK7(+)/CK20(−)/CDX-2(−) is a typical pattern for EMC, while CK7(−)/CK20(+)/CDX-2(+) be for colorectal cancer.

5.3.5 Tumorigenesis and Genetic Background (Fig. 5.1)

Endometriosis is considered to be a precursor of EMC, particularly the low-grade. The recent analysis of molecular genetic changes shared by both endometriosis and EMC supports the tumorigenesis, in that it is suggested that most EMCs are caused by malignant transformation of endometriosis and may not derive from ovarian surface epithelium [45–48]. Endometrioid borderline/atypical proliferative endometrioid tumor also has the genetic changes which are common in endometriosis. While the tumorigenesis of high-grade EMC has yet to be clarified, many of them are recently regarded as high-grade SEC with glandular differentiation. Some of the high-grade EMCs are supposed to have developed from low-grade EMC due to the existence of molecular changes common in both low-grade and high-grade EMCs, such as *TP53* mutation [1, 49]. The frequent association of ovarian EMC with endometriosis, endometrial carcinoma, or both of them suggests that ovarian EMC may share the same risk factors as endometrial carcinoma [50].

PTEN and PIK3CA: The tumor suppressor gene of *PTEN*, located in chromosome 10q23.3, is inactivated by its mutations in 14–21% of EMCs [47, 51]. *PTEN* inactivation may be caused by several mechanisms such as mutation, loss of heterozygosity (LOH) at 10q23, and promoter hypermethylation and encodes a lipid phosphatase which antagonizes PI3K/Akt pathway by dephosphorylating PIP_3, the product of PI3K. The mutations of *PIK3CA*, mainly clustered in exons 9 and 20, are identified in up to 20% of EMCs [52] and are adverse prognostic parameters. *PIK3CA* and *PTEN* mutations co-occur [53, 54], and an additive effect on the PI3K pathway has been suggested [2, 55]. The majority of EMCs with *PTEN* mutation are well differentiated and stage I, suggesting that *PTEN* inactivation is an early event in this subset of ovarian tumors [2, 47, 51, 56].

CTNNB1: β-Catenin-mediated canonical Wnt pathway signaling goes through a dysregulation in 16–38% of EMCs [54, 57–60]. Several studies have reported the association of *CTNNB1* mutation with squamous differentiation, low-grade and favorable outcome [53, 54, 56, 61].

ARID1A: Inactivated mutations of *ARID1A*, which encodes a subunit of the SWI/SNF chromatin remodeling

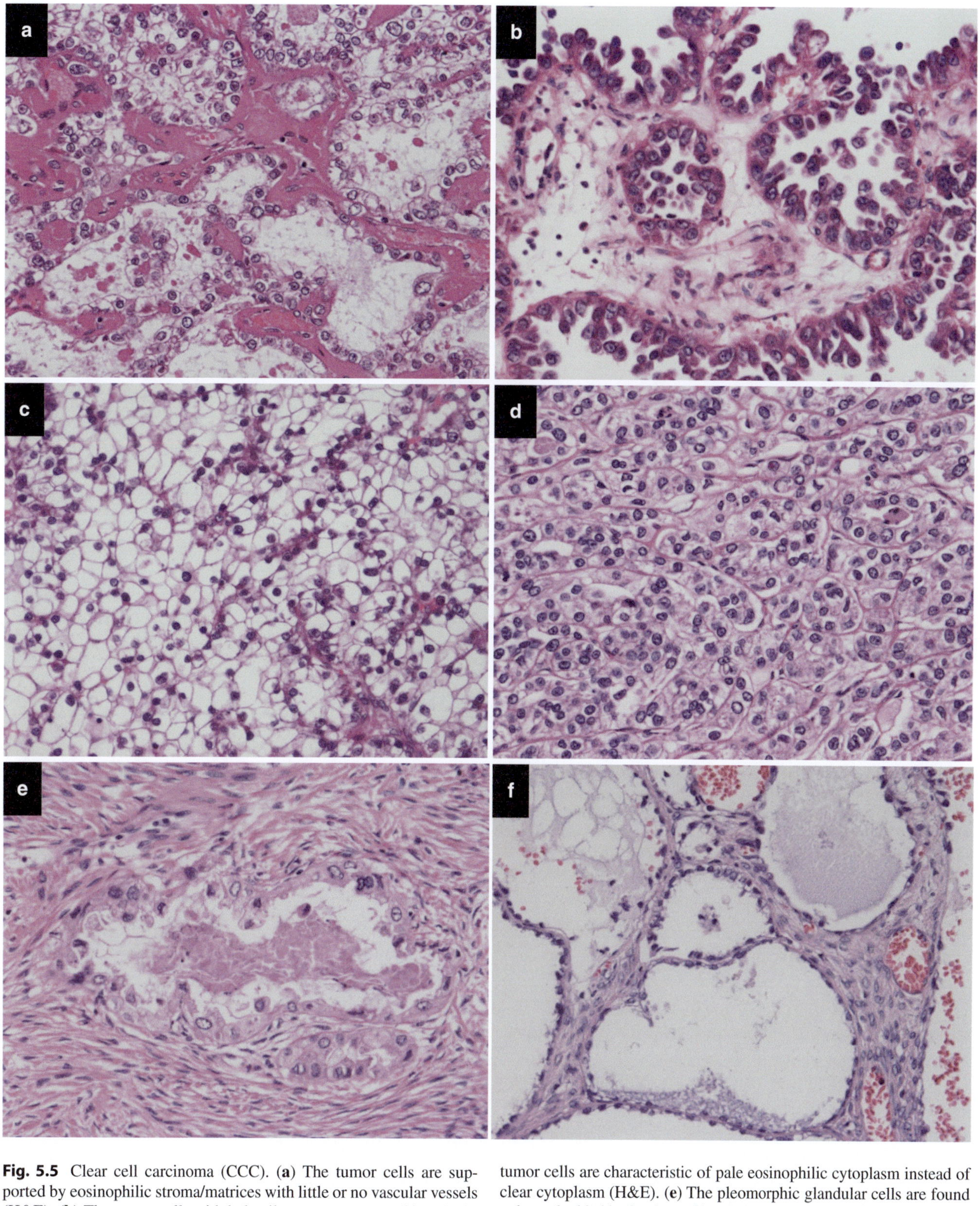

Fig. 5.5 Clear cell carcinoma (CCC). (**a**) The tumor cells are supported by eosinophilic stroma/matrices with little or no vascular vessels (H&E). (**b**) The tumor cells with hobnail appearance are tufting, looking detached in the glandular lumen (H&E). (**c**) Solid nests are composed of the tumor cells with abundant clear cytoplasm (H&E). (**d**) The tumor cells are characteristic of pale eosinophilic cytoplasm instead of clear cytoplasm (H&E). (**e**) The pleomorphic glandular cells are found to be embedded in the dense fibrotic stroma, categorized into adenocarcinofibroma type (H&E). (**f**) The tubulocystic nests are lined by flattened atypical clear cells in a single-layered manner (H&E)

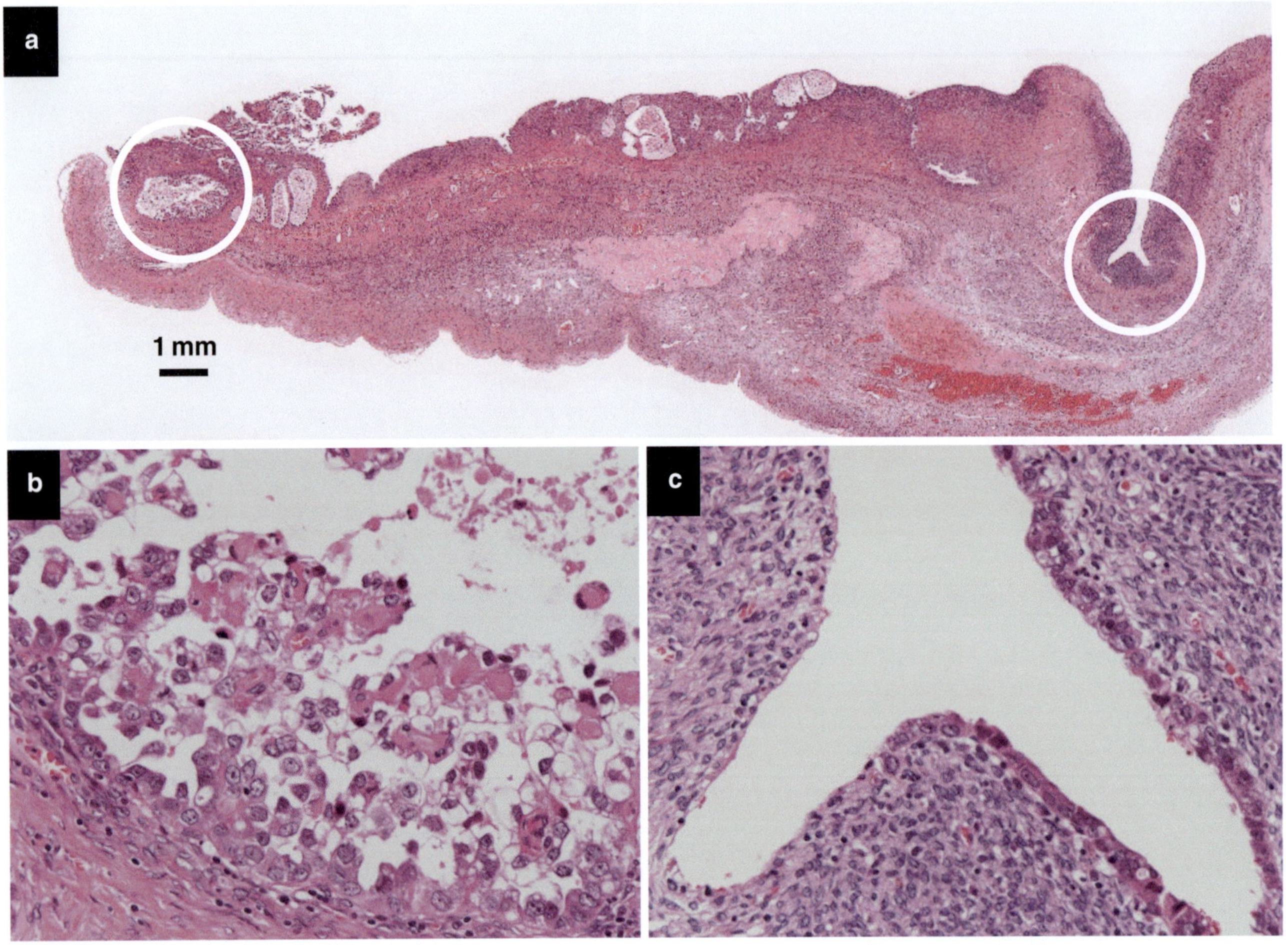

Fig. 5.6 Clear cell carcinoma (CCC) in an early stage (incidentally detected small lesions in the endometriotic cyst). (**a**) The loupe view shows multiple small foci of the tumor cells in the cystic wall with a background of atypical endometriosis (H&E). (**b**) The tumor cells are highly atypical, producing eosinophilic matrix with occasional hyaline globular appearance (H&E). (**c**) The atypical cells are arranged in a single or a few layers, supported by endometrial stroma-like cells, identical to atypical endometriosis (H&E). (**d**) The tumor cells are positive for HNF-1β in the nuclei (immunohistochemistry). (**e**) The nuclei of atypical endometriosis are also positively labeled by HNF-1β (immunohistochemistry). (**f**) No positive reaction of ARID1A is observed in the nuclei of tumor cells (immunohistochemistry). (**g**) No positive reaction of ARID1A is observed in the nuclei of atypical endometriosis (immunohistochemistry)

complex, take place in 30% of EMC [62], resulting in function loss of *ARID1A* typically due to frameshift or nonsense mutations.

TP53: The mutations have been reported in 60% of EMCs arising in the ovary, most often in high-grade EMCs. Along with the high prevalence of *TP53* mutations in high-grade SECs, it is supposed that many previously diagnosed high-grade EMC, categorized as grade 3, might be more appropriately reclassified as high-grade SEC [63–65]. Mutations typical of low-grade EMC are not usually shared by high-grade EMC, suggesting that it is difficult to discriminate between high-grade EMC and high-grade SEC based on the genetic profiles [54, 66].

MLH1 and *MSH2*: Occasional cases with EMC develop in families with germline mutations in DNA mismatch repair gems such as *MLH1* and *MSH2*, called Muir-Torre syndrome [67], which is thought to be a variant of the hereditary nonpolyposis colon cancer syndrome [68]. Microsatellite instability is observed in 13–20% of EMCs [51, 69]. Activated mutations in *KRAS* and *BRAF* may occur in EMC [54, 70–73].

Methylenetetrahydrofolate dehydrogenase 1 (MTHFD1) and estrogen receptor (ER), which are expressed in endometrial secretory cells, show the higher expression in EMC than CCC. But, CTH is strongly expressed in ciliated cells, not only in CCC but also in eutopic endometrium, endometriosis, and the fallopian tube. It is proposed that the specific ciliated or secretory cellular contexts may provide an explanation for how endometriosis may give rise to both EMC and CCC [18].

5.3.6 Prognostic Considerations

EMC of the ovary associated with the endometrial EMC occurs in 15–20% of cases [21, 22, 74, 75]. Usually, both

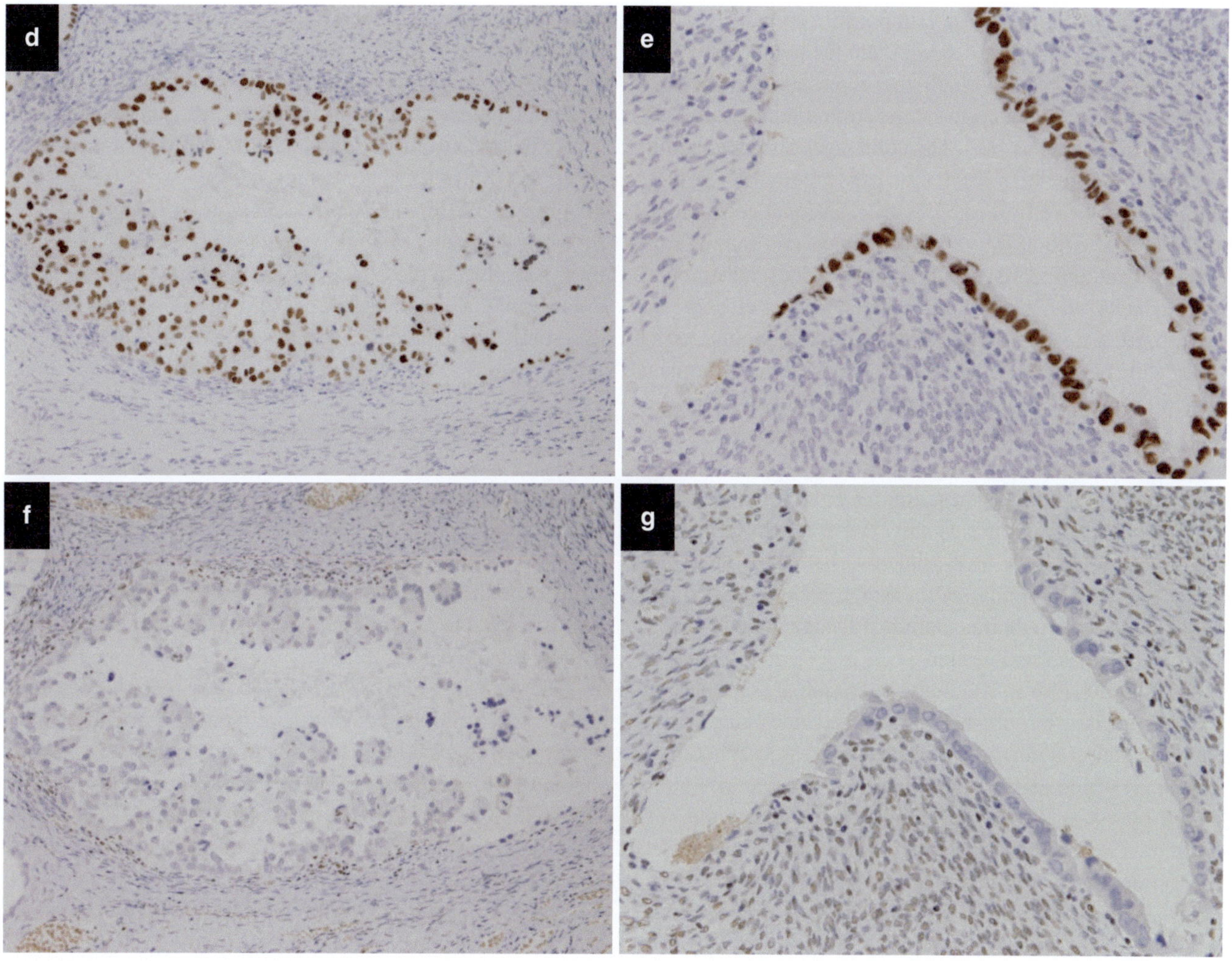

Fig. 5.6 (continued)

tumors are well differentiated and resemble each other. The criteria for discrimination between metastatic EMC and primary EMC in the ovary depend on the clinicopathological features. When the endometrial EMC is low-grade and associated with hyperplasia and shows little or no myometrial invasion, an independency of the ovarian EMC can be warranted to a large extent. Then, the association of ovarian EMC with endometriosis, adenofibroma, or endometrioid borderline tumor/atypical proliferative endometrioid tumor is also suggestive of the independency of the ovarian EMC from endometrial EMC. These interpretations are supported by the following evidence with the patients' prognosis: the 5-year survival is 70–92%; the median survival is 10 years or longer [9, 76]; and most of the patients survive without recurrence [74, 77, 78]. However, when the ovarian EMC is bilateral and the endometrial EMC deeply invades the myometrium with obvious lymphovascular invasions, it is more likely that the ovarian EMC is to be metastasizing from the endometrial EMC.

5.4 Clear Cell Carcinoma (Figs. 5.5 and 5.6)

5.4.1 Gross

The majorities of CCCs are confined to the unilateral ovary with a mean size of 15 cm and are composed of solid and cystic parts to variable extents [79–82]. The solid parts of the carcinoma may represent a background of benign (adenofibroma) and/or borderline tumor. CCC typically is composed of endometriotic cystic lesion in the background, containing fleshy pale yellow parts [83], but not infrequently takes the form of a cyst alone composed of a thickened wall.

5.4.2 Histopathology (Figs. 5.5 and 5.6)

The carcinoma cells of CCC, which are characterized by the production of glycogen, are arranged in papillary, solid, and tubulocystic nests, and these components are admixed in a variable pattern [83, 84]. Among them the most characteristic are the papillae, of which the cores are composed of amorphous or acellular eosinophilic stroma/matrix with little or no vascular vessels [85]. The solid nests are separated by fine septa. The nuclei of carcinoma cells are round to polygonal, and eccentrically located, with occasional conspicuous nucleoli. The cytoplasm varies in amount and ranges from clear to eosinophilic. Especially in the tubulocystic structure, hobnail cells with apical hyperchromatic nuclei and relatively narrow clear cytoplasm project into the luminal cavity. Cells with high-grade nuclei and/or those with prominent nucleoli are usually admixed with cells with low-grade or even bland nuclear features [86]. Intracytoplasmic or extracytoplasmic hyaline globular secretions are sometimes observed. The mitotic figures, ranging from mean 3 to 4 per 10 high-power fields, are usually less frequently observed than in serous or other high-grade ovarian carcinomas [86]. The clear or eosinophilic cytoplasm contains PAS-positive fine granules due to their containing glycogen which is demonstrated by diastase digestion.

CCC, which is grossly mainly composed of homogeneous solid parts, is often characteristic of adenocarcinofibroma with relatively abundant fibrotic stroma or rarely functioning stroma, in which production of sex steroid hormones represented by estrogen (mainly estradiol) is encountered. The carcinoma is to a less or more extent accompanied with clear cell borderline/atypical proliferative clear cell tumor and clear adenofibroma (Fig. 5.7). The glands in clear cell borderline/atypical proliferative clear cell tumor are typically round to oval and relatively evenly spaced in a fibromatous stroma. Compacted glands with stromal reaction may be invasive. The cells lining cysts and glands are cuboidal, hobnail, or flattened cells but are less atypical, compared to carcinoma cells with infrequent mitotic figs [79, 82, 87].

There is no established grading system for CCC because of the recognition that all of the CCCs are high-grade carcinoma, irrespective of a wide range of histological differentiation. In case of CCC containing very poorly differentiated histology, solid masses or individual cells infiltrating with little or no glandular/papillary differentiate in >5% [88] or at least 10% [89] of the tumor; the prognosis is supposed to be unfavorable, compared to the tumor composed of well-differentiated tubulocystic and/or papillary architecture.

5.4.3 Differential Diagnoses

Serous carcinoma (SEC): Papillary architecture and hobnail appearance are often in common with SEC. CCC and SEC develops papillary trunk containing vascular vessels, but fine papillae with little stromal core and slit-like narrow spaces found in solid nests are limited to SEC. Hobnail cells in SEC usually have scant cytoplasm.

Endometrioid carcinoma (EMC): Eosinophilic type of CCC mimics EMC. Recognition of typical clear cell components, even to a minor extent, may be a useful hallmark for distinguishing CCC from EMC. Papillary architecture with eosinophilic core supports the diagnosis of CCC. On the other hand, in the case with squamous differentiation, EMC is more favorable (Fig. 5.3).

Yolk sac tumor (YST): The tumor cells of YST also have clear cytoplasm, and take variable morphological patterns, of which some are specific for YST but others are not. Call-Exner bodies may be diagnostically reliable. Hyaline globules with PAS-positive reaction are often found in both CCC

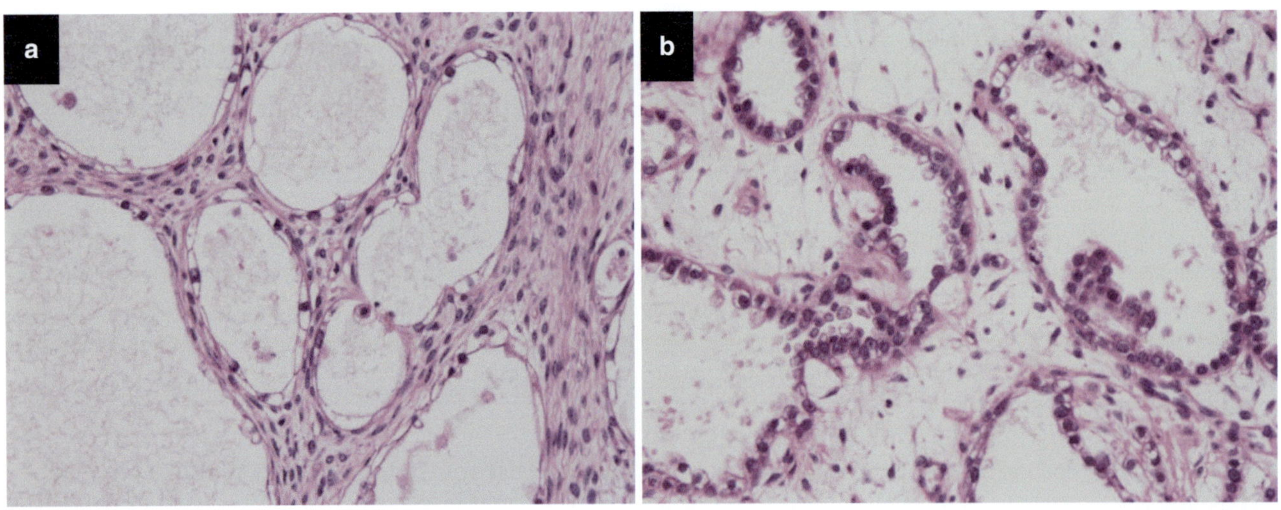

Fig. 5.7 Clear cell borderline tumor. (**a**) The cuboidal tumor cells possess mildly atypical nuclei and clear cytoplasm (H&E). (**b**) The enlarged tumor cells show hobnail appearance and less abundant clear cytoplasm (H&E)

and YST. The patient age and prominent serum elevation of alpha-fetoprotein (AFP) value are helpful for the diagnostic confirmation of both tumors.

Metastatic renal clear cell carcinoma: Refer to Sect. 5.4.4.

5.4.4 Immunohistochemistry (Fig. 5.6)

Hepatocellular nuclear factor (HNF)-1β: As long as YST is excluded, HNF-1β is observed to be expressed in 80% of CCCs diffusely and strongly as a specific marker [90–92]. But, HNF-1β is also expressed in mid- to late-secretory phase endometrium, suggesting the association with physio-pathological cytoplasmic glycogen accumulation [91].

ARID1A: The function loss of ARID1A due to the mutation often occurs. Thus, many CCCs are immunohistochemically negative for the antibody which reacts with the wild-type ARID1A. Loss of ARID1A expression is mostly associated with *PIK3CA* mutations [86].

Napsin-A: This antigen has been known as a specific marker of lung adenocarcinoma because of the involvement of maturation of surfactant protein B. Among the ovarian carcinomas, Napsin-A is helpful in differentiation of CCC with high sensitivity and specificity from other carcinomas [93, 94].

AFP: In comparison with other markers, AFP is almost confined to YST, some of which has been reported to arise from somatic adenocarcinoma, represented by EMC [95, 96]. In CCC, focal expression of AFP may be encountered [38].

Spalt-like transcriptional factor 4 (SALL4) and glypican-3 (GPC3): When distinguishing CCC from germ cell tumors represented by YST, SALL4 of zinc finger transcription factor is helpful. SALL4 is a stem cell marker which is reactivated in variable cancers. But, it should be noted that some CCCs may show a positive reaction. GPC3, i.e., placental and fetal hepatic heparin sulfate proteoglycan, is an oncofetal protein which is used as one of the germ cell tumor markers. Incorporation of SALL4 with other panels such as AFP and GPC3 is practically significant in differentiation between CCC and YST [97, 98].

Estrogen receptor (ER) and progesterone receptor (PgR): More than 90% of CCCs show minimally positive or negative reaction [99, 100].

CK7 and CD10: Diffuse strong positive reaction for CK7 and absence of CD10 favor the ovarian CCC, and renal cell carcinoma antigen is also helpful. However, it should be noted that both ovarian and renal CCCs express HNF-1β and Pax-8.

5.4.5 Tumorigenesis and Genetic Background (Fig. 5.1)

There are two distinct histogenetic pathways as follows: most of the CCCs occur in association with endometriosis [62]; the minorities are considered to arise from clear cell borderline tumor/atypical proliferative clear cell tumor, and adjacent atypical endometriosis, supporting endometriosis as the precursor [62, 101].

ARID1A, PIK3CA, and PTEN: The most representative mutated genes identified in CCC include *ARID1A* in 46–57% [62, 102], *PIK3CA* in 40% [52, 103, 104], and *PTEN* in 8.3% [48]. *ARID1A* somatic inactivated mutations correlate with loss of BAF250a, which is encoded by *ARID1A* [62, 102]. *ARID1A* mutation and BAF250a loss are also identified in the adjacent endometriotic lesions but not in those distant from CCC [62]. *PIK3CA*-activated mutations are closely linked with *ARID1A*-deficient carcinomas [105]. These cooperated gene mutations are supposed to occur as an early event during the tumorigenesis. When clear cell borderline tumor/atypical proliferative clear cell tumor coexists with CCC, they share genetic abnormalities such as *ARID1A* mutation, indicating that these tumors are clonally related [88, 105, 106] and have a similar immunoprofiles [82].

MSH2: CCC is associated with Lynch syndrome, most commonly in association with germline mutations in *MSH2* [107–111], but not with hereditary ovarian-breast cancer syndrome (e.g., *BRCA1* or *BRCA2* mutation).

The certain endometriosis-associated genetic mutations are shared by CCC and EMC, and it is unique that the differences in the genomic landscape features between EMC and CCC are not absolute. The issue about how endometriosis leads to the two distinct histologic types remains to be clarified. The specific expression of CTH in CCC, but not in EMC, suggests its derivation from ciliated cells of endometriosis (refer to Sect. 5.3.5).

5.4.6 Prognostic Considerations

CCCs staged IC due to intraoperative rupture shows the same prognosis as those staged IA, and the prognosis of all other stage IC is similar to that of stage II CCCs [23, 112]. Poor responsiveness to platinum-based chemotherapy has been shown in high-stage tumors, resulting in poor overall and disease-specific survival [3, 5, 113]. CCCs with adenofibromatous components may be a distinct subgroup because of the less aggressive biological behavior [114]. In the background of the speculation, there has been the presence of two distinct tumorigenetic pathways to the ovarian CCC: allelic status of clear cell adenofibroma is supposed to show a clonal precursor of CCC [106, 115]. Newly proposed grading schemes, based on the occupation ratios of well-differentiated and poorly differentiated CCC components, are as follows: group A, 90% or more is well differentiated; group C, 10% or more is poorly differentiated; and group B, all other CCCs [89]. The 5-year survivals are 100% for A, 82% for B, and

56% for C in CCCs staged I and II and 48% for A, 51% for B, and 16% for C in CCCs staged III and IV.

Paraneoplastic hypercalcemia [116] and venous thromboembolism [117–119] are most closely complicated with CCC. It is also associated with Lynch syndrome [107–111]. *PIK3CA* mutations [120] and *PIK3CA* overexpression [121] are found to be correlated with improved survival. In contrast, loss of ARID1A expression is correlated with shorter progression-free survival and chemoresistance [122].

5.5 Seromucinous Tumors (Figs. 5.8 and 5.9)

There are three subclasses of seromucinous tumors: seromucinous cystadenoma/adenofibroma (synonym, müllerian cystadenoma of mixed cell types), seromucinous borderline tumor/atypical proliferative seromucinous tumor (synonym, endocervical-type mucinous borderline tumor, müllerian mucinous borderline tumor, atypical proliferative (borderline) müllerian tumor), and seromucinous carcinoma (synonym, endocervical-type mucinous and mixed epithelial carcinomas of müllerian type). In terms of the tumorigenesis, the association with endometriosis is common in all of these tumors.

5.5.1 Seromucinous Cystadenoma/Adenofibroma

A benign cystic lesion, characterized by coexistence of two or more müllerian cell types accounting for at least 10% of benign ovarian tumors, is typically present as a unilocular cyst containing serous or mucinous fluid. Histopathologically,

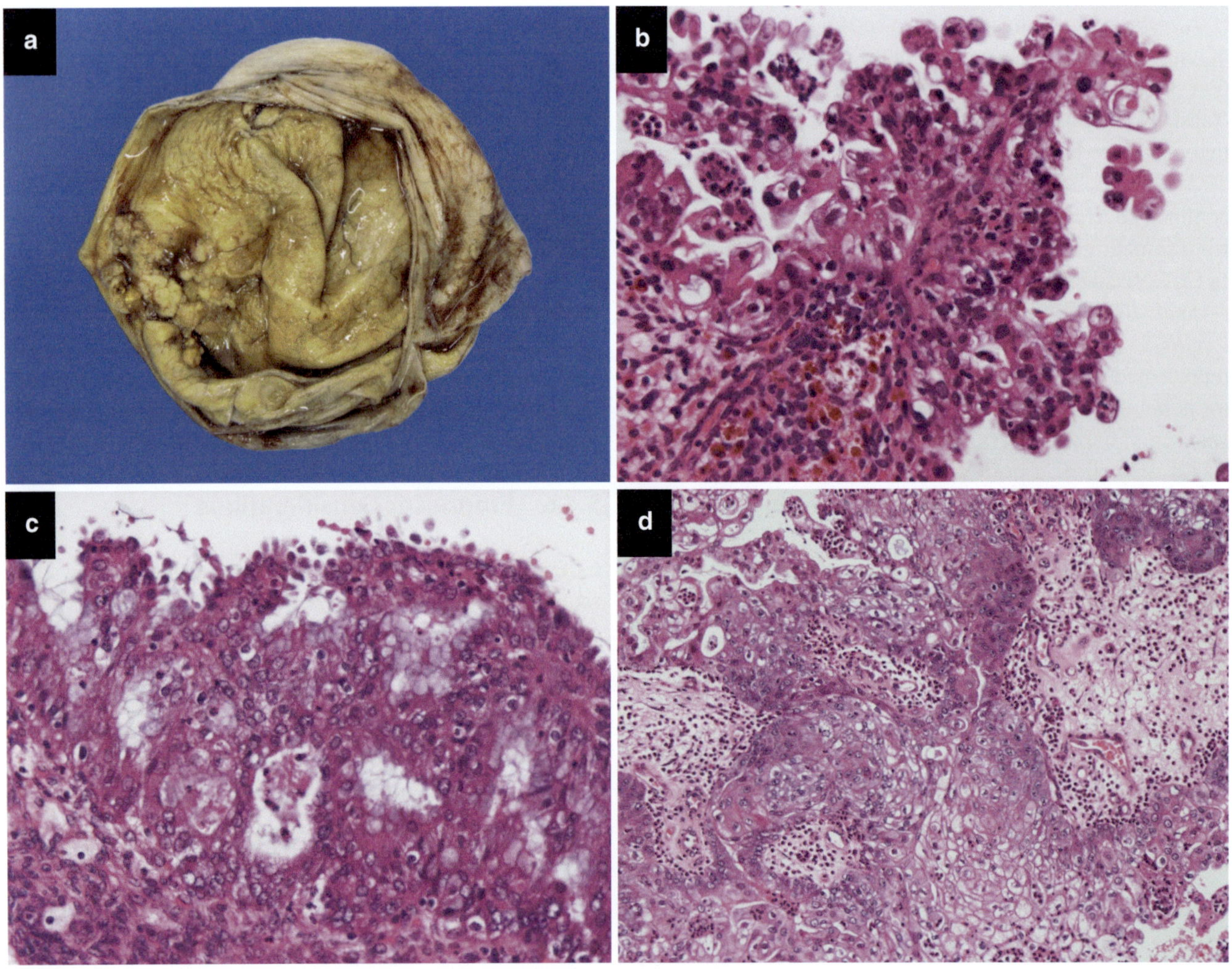

Fig. 5.8 Seromucinous borderline tumor. (**a**) The loupe view shows solid and elevated components, mimicking serous borderline tumor. (**b**) The tumor cells are stratified with papillary pattern, composed of cells with mixed serous and mucinous cells (H&E). (**c**) Mucin-producing cells are arranged in a tubular manner, covered by cells with hobnail appearance in the surface (H&E). (**d**) The gland-forming tumor cells are differentiated into well-differentiated squamous cells (H&E)

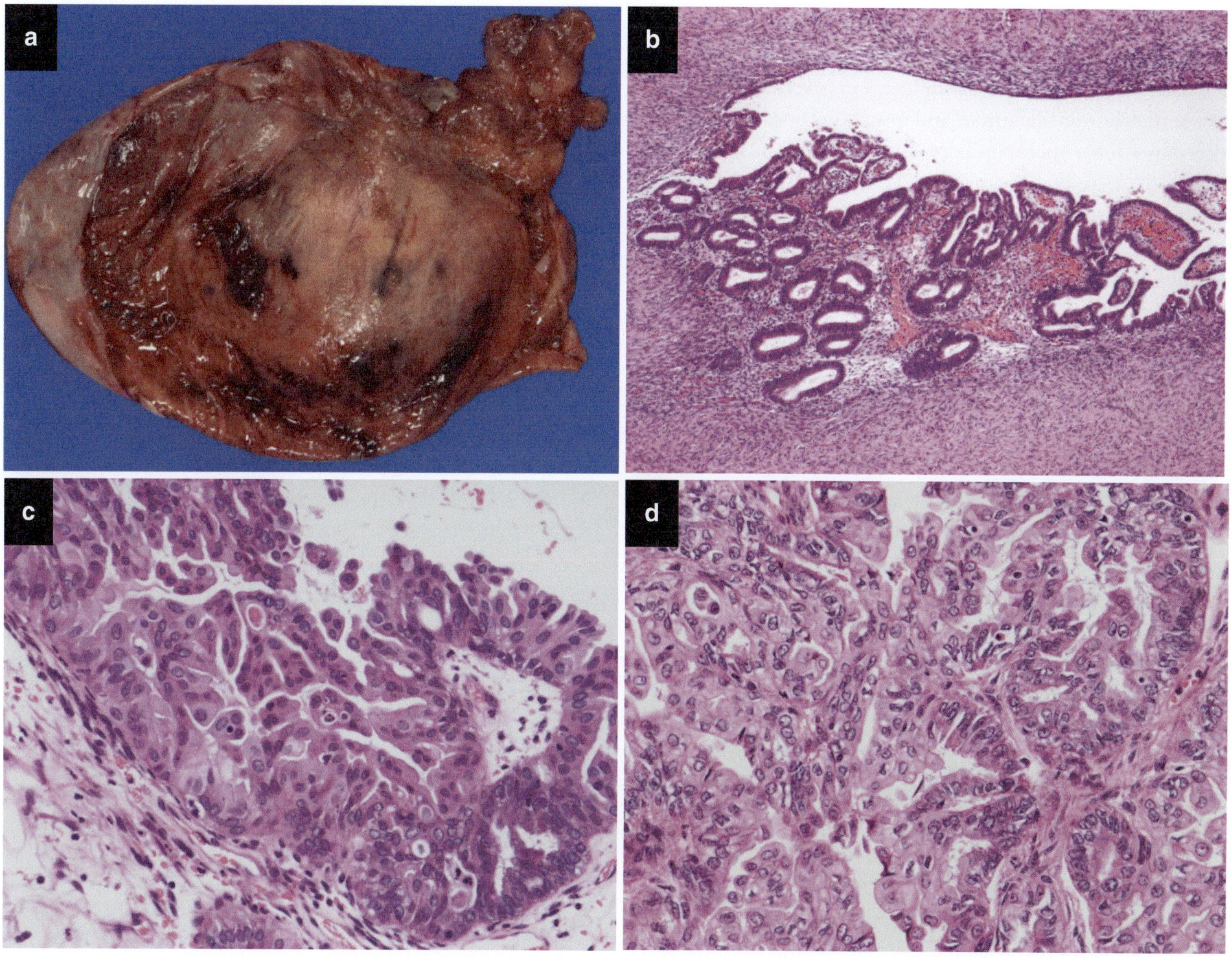

Fig. 5.9 Seromucinous carcinoma. (**a**) The gross view shows a cystic lesion containing a papillary-protruding tumor and hemorrhagic area. (**b**) Ectopic endometrial tissues are present in the background (H&E). (**c**) Papillary parts are composed of mixed serous and mucinous cells, arranged in stratified papillary manner (H&E). (**d**) Complex and crowded glands with squamous differentiation are showing invasive proliferation (H&E)

the cysts are lined by a variable admixture of mainly serous and mucinous cells (endocervical type), and less often endometrioid or squamous cells may be seen.

5.5.2 Seromucinous Borderline Tumor/Atypical Proliferative Seromucinous Tumor (Fig. 5.8)

Until recently, this tumor had been considered to be a subset of mucinous tumors, known as endocervical type, accounting for 15% of mucinous borderline tumors [123]. The tumorigenesis is not related to borderline/atypical proliferative mucinous tumors, gastrointestinal type. Mucinous cells of the endocervical type with mild to moderate atypia are the main components, with coexistence of serous and other epithelial types such as endometrioid, clear cell, and transitional or squamous cells. The patients are aged 34–44 years [123–127]. The tumorigenesis is associated with endometriosis in about a third of the cases [128]. The majority of patients are staged I, but a minority are advanced in stage due to implants and/or lymph node involvement.

The tumor is typically unilateral but bilateral in up to 40%, measuring 8–10 cm in diameter [123–127], and occupied by variable-sized friable papillary excrescences in the cyst with a viscid fluid. The association with endometriosis is indicated by granular to hemorrhagic foci. Histopathologically, the tumor architecturally resembles serous borderline/atypical proliferative serous tumor [129], represented by complex papillary or branching architecture in a hierarchical manner. The smaller papillae terminate with small detached epithelial tufts, and the larger papillae are edematous in the stroma with neutrophilic infiltrates. The surface of these papillae is lined by stratified cells of mostly endocervical-type mucinous or serous epithelium. Endometrioid and squamous or clear cells are often seen.

The cytoplasm is often eosinophilic, and the nuclear atypia is in a low-grade. Mitotic figures are infrequently observed. There is no presence of destructive, i.e., overt, invasion, but like serous borderline tumor and mucinous borderline tumor, microinvasion, micropapillary features and intraepithelial carcinoma may be encountered [124, 125, 127, 130]. In the background, the lining cells mimic uterine endometrial glandular cells with occasional underlying proper stromal cells. Immunohistochemically, these tumors usually express ER and PgR [131–133].

Endometrial-type tissue may undergo mucinous metaplasia, which then sequentially evolves into a cystadenoma and a borderline/atypical proliferative tumor [1, 134]. The association with endometriosis, ER positivity and lack of WT-1 expression, suggests a close relationship to endometrioid and clear cell neoplasms [128, 132], which is further supported by the finding of *ARID1A* mutations and loss of expression in a proportion of these tumors similar to EMC and CCC [128]. Function loss of ARID1A, occurring in one third of the tumors, is similar to EMC and CCCs in the frequency [128]. Even with the peritoneal implants, the tumor shows a good outcome [123–127].

5.5.3 Seromucinous Carcinoma (Fig. 5.9)

Previously, seromucinous carcinoma in the current terminology in the WHO 2003 classification was designated as endocervical-like mucinous carcinoma. According to the WHO 2014 classification, the carcinoma cells are predominantly serous and endocervical-type mucinous, occasionally containing foci of clear cells and endometrioid cells with squamous differentiation [135]. This tumor is generally low-grade with favorable prognosis and tends to be diagnosed at a younger age and at a low stage, compared to SEC [135, 136]. The mean age is 45 years old [127].

The mean tumor size is 12 cm, and more than half of the tumors show bilaterality [127]. The tumors are unilocular or multilocular and contain variable amounts of solid areas or papillary excrescences in the cyst and/or on the surface. Histopathologically, tumors cells commonly show papillary stratification closely resembling serous tumors and are arranged in a confluent or expansile invasive manner with a cribriform structure. These tumors contain endocervical-type mucinous and serous-type epithelium, but cells with clear cytoplasm, not displaying patterns of CCC, as well as foci of endometrioid differentiation, including squamous cells may also be present [127]. The mitotic index is variable but tends to be low: less than 5 mitotic figures per 10 high-power fields. The immunohistochemical profile is similar to the borderline/atypical proliferative group of seromucinous tumors. Parenthetically, it should be noted that besides seromucinous carcinomas which can show a variety of cell types, all the epithelial ovarian tumors can also show mixtures of cell types. They are classified by the predominant type, but the smaller components can be included in the diagnosis. For example, a high-grade serous carcinoma with an endometrioid component showing clear-cut squamous differentiation could be classified as a "high-grade serous carcinoma with endometrioid differentiation."

The tumorigenesis remains to be clarified because of the small number of reported cases, with which the poor reproducibility is a diagnostic problem [24]. In particular, the distinction of seromucinous carcinoma from endometrioid carcinoma with mucinous differentiation and low-grade serous carcinoma can be arbitrary [24, 136]. The molecular features overlap mostly with endometrioid and low-grade serous carcinomas: the prevalence of target gene mutations is 70% for *KRAS*, 37% for *PIK3CA*, 29% for *PTEN*, 16% for *ARID1A*, and 0% for *CTNNB1* [136]. In terms of the frequent coexistence with seromucinous borderline/atypical proliferative tumors (Fig. 5.8) and endometriosis, it is likely that endometriosis is the precursor lesion. The outcome of patients staged I is favorable, but half of the patients with advanced-stage tumors died of disease [127].

References

1. Kurman RJ, Carcangiu ML, Herrington CS, Young BH, and editors. Chapter 1: Tumours of the ovary. In: World Health Organization Classification of Tumours of Female Reproductive Organs. Lyon: IARC; 2014.
2. Mutter GL, Prat J, and editors. Chapter 27: Ovarian endometrioid, clear cell, transitional, and mixed epithelial stromal tumor. In: Pathology of the female reproductive tract. 3rd ed. London: Churchill Livingstone Elsevier; 2014.
3. Chan JK, Teoh D, Hu JM, Shin JY, Osann K, Kapp DS. Do clear cell ovarian carcinomas have poorer prognosis compared to other epithelial cell types? A study of 1411 clear cell ovarian cancers. Gynecol Oncol. 2008;109(3):370–6.
4. Itamochi H, Kigawa J, Terakawa N. Mechanisms of chemoresistance and poor prognosis in ovarian clear cell carcinoma. Cancer Sci. 2008;99(4):653–8.
5. Sugiyama T, Kamura T, Kigawa J, Terakawa N, Kikuchi Y, Kita T, Suzuki M, Sato I, Taguchi K. Clinical characteristics of clear cell carcinoma of the ovary: a distinct histologic type with poor prognosis and resistance to platinum-based chemotherapy. Cancer. 2000;88(11):2584–9.
6. Kennedy AW, Biscotti CV, Hart WR, Webster KD. Ovarian clear cell adenocarcinoma. Gynecol Oncol. 1989;32(3):342–9.
7. Aure JC, Hoeg K, Kolstad P. Clinical and histologic studies of ovarian carcinoma. Long-term follow-up of 990 cases. Obstet Gynecol. 1971;37(1):1–9.
8. Scully RE, Young RH, Clement PB. Tumor of ovary, maldeveloped gonads, fallopian tube, and broad ligament. In: Atlas of tumor pathology, 3rd ed. Third series. Fascicle 23. Washington, DC: Armed Forces Institute of Pathology; 1998. p. 153–164.
9. Storey DJ, Rush R, Stewart M, Rye T, Al-Nafussi A, Williams AR, Smyth JF, Gabra H. Endometrioid epithelial ovarian cancer : 20 years of prospectively collected data from a single center. Cancer. 2008;112(10):2211–20.

10. Bell KA, Kurman RJ. A clinicopathologic analysis of atypical proliferative (borderline) tumors and well-differentiated endometrioid adenocarcinomas of the ovary. Am J Surg Pathol. 2000;24(11):1465–79.
11. Pettersson F. Annual report of the results of treatment in gynecological cancer. Stockholm: International Federation of Gynecology and Obstetrics; 1991.
12. Aoki D. Annual Report of Gynecologic Oncology Committee, Japan Society of Obstetrics and Gynecology, 2013. J Obstet Gynaecol Res. 2014;40(2):338–48.
13. DePriest PD, Banks ER, Powell DE, van Nagell JR Jr, Gallion HH, Puls LE, Hunter JE, Kryscio RJ, Royalty MB. Endometrioid carcinoma of the ovary and endometriosis: the association in postmenopausal women. Gynecol Oncol. 1992;47(1):71–5.
14. Mostoufizadeh M, Scully RE. Malignant tumors arising in endometriosis. Clin Obstet Gynecol. 1980;23(3):951–63.
15. McMeekin DS, Burger RA, Manetta A, DiSaia P, Berman ML. Endometrioid adenocarcinoma of the ovary and its relationship to endometriosis. Gynecol Oncol. 1995;59(1):81–6.
16. Fukunaga M, Nomura K, Ishikawa E, Ushigome S. Ovarian atypical endometriosis: its close association with malignant epithelial tumours. Histopathology. 1997;30(3):249–55.
17. Ogawa S, Kaku T, Amada S, Kobayashi H, Hirakawa T, Ariyoshi K, Kamura T, Nakano H. Ovarian endometriosis associated with ovarian carcinoma: a clinicopathological and immunohistochemical study. Gynecol Oncol. 2000;77(2):298–304.
18. Cochrane DR, Tessier-Cloutier B, Lawrence KM, Nazeran T, Karnezis AN, Salamanca C, Cheng AS, McAlpine JN, Hoang LN, Gilks CB, Huntsman DG. Clear cell and endometrioid carcinomas: are their differences attributable to distinct cells of origin? J Pathol. 2017;243(1):26–36.
19. Pearce CL, Templeman C, Rossing MA, Lee A, Near AM, Webb PM, Nagle CM, Doherty JA, Cushing-Haugen KL, Wicklund KG, Chang-Claude J, Hein R, Lurie G, Wilkens LR, Carney ME, Goodman MT, Moysich K, Kjaer SK, Hogdall E, Jensen A, Goode EL, Fridley BL, Larson MC, Schildkraut JM, Palmieri RT, Cramer DW, Terry KL, Vitonis AF, Titus LJ, Ziogas A, Brewster W, Anton-Culver H, Gentry-Maharaj A, Ramus SJ, Anderson AR, Brueggmann D, Fasching PA, Gayther SA, Huntsman DG, Menon U, Ness RB, Pike MC, Risch H, Wu AH, Berchuck A. Association between endometriosis and risk of histological subtypes of ovarian cancer: a pooled analysis of case-control studies. Lancet Oncol. 2012;13(4):385–94.
20. Irving JA, Catasus L, Gallardo A, Bussaglia E, Romero M, Matias-Guiu X, Prat J. Synchronous endometrioid carcinomas of the uterine corpus and ovary: alterations in the beta-catenin (CTNNB1) pathway are associated with independent primary tumors and favorable prognosis. Hum Pathol. 2005;36(6):605–19.
21. Kline RC, Wharton JT, Atkinson EN, Burke TW, Gershenson DM, Edwards CL. Endometrioid carcinoma of the ovary: retrospective review of 145 cases. Gynecol Oncol. 1990;39(3):337–46.
22. Zaino RJ, Unger ER, Whitney C. Synchronous carcinomas of the uterine corpus and ovary. Gynecol Oncol. 1984;19(3):329–35.
23. Higashi M, Kajiyama H, Shibata K, Mizuno M, Mizuno K, Hosono S, Kawai M, Nakanishi T, Nagasaka T, Kikkawa F. Survival impact of capsule rupture in stage I clear cell carcinoma of the ovary in comparison with other histological types. Gynecol Oncol. 2011;123(3):474–8.
24. Rutgers JL. Mullerian mucinous/mixed epithelial (seromucinous) ovarian tumors. Am J Surg Pathol Rev Rep. 2016;21:206–13.
25. Kurman RJ, Shih IM. Molecular pathogenesis and extraovarian origin of epithelial ovarian cancer—shifting the paradigm. Hum Pathol. 2011;42(7):918–31.
26. Bulun SE. Endometriosis. N Engl J Med. 2009;360(3):268–79.
27. Rosenblatt KA, Thomas DB. Reduced risk of ovarian cancer in women with a tubal ligation or hysterectomy. The World Health Organization collaborative study of neoplasia and steroid contraceptives. Cancer Epidemiol Biomark Prev. 1996;5(11):933–5.
28. Burney RO, Giudice LC. Pathogenesis and pathophysiology of endometriosis. Fertil Steril. 2012;98(3):511–9.
29. Mutter GL, Prat J, and editors. Chapter 22: Endometriosis. In: Pathology of the female reproductive tract. 3rd ed. London: Churchill Livingstone Elsevier; 2014.
30. Eskenazi B, Warner ML. Epidemiology of endometriosis. Obstet Gynecol Clin N Am. 1997;24(2):235–58.
31. Sangi-Haghpeykar H, Poindexter AN III. Epidemiology of endometriosis among parous women. Obstet Gynecol. 1995;85(6):983–92.
32. Vessey MP, Villard-Mackintosh L, Painter R. Epidemiology of endometriosis in women attending family planning clinics. BMJ. 1993;306(6871):182–4.
33. Anglesio MS, Papadopoulos N, Ayhan A, Nazeran TM, Noe M, Horlings HM, Lum A, Jones S, Senz J, Seckin T, Ho J, Wu RC, Lac V, Ogawa H, Tessier-Cloutier B, Alhassan R, Wang A, Wang Y, Cohen JD, Wong F, Hasanovic A, Orr N, Zhang M, Popoli M, McMahon W, Wood LD, Mattox A, Allaire C, Segars J, Williams C, Tomasetti C, Boyd N, Kinzler KW, Gilks CB, Diaz L, Wang TL, Vogelstein B, Yong PJ, Huntsman DG, Shih IM. Cancer-associated mutations in endometriosis without Cancer. N Engl J Med. 2017;376(19):1835–48.
34. Creasman WT, Odicino F, Maisonneuve P, Quinn MA, Beller U, Benedet JL, Heintz AP, Ngan HY, Pecorelli S. Carcinoma of the corpus uteri. FIGO 26th annual report on the results of treatment in gynecological cancer. Int J Gynaecol Obstet. 2006;95(Suppl 1):S105–43.
35. Brescia RJ, Dubin N, Demopoulos RI. Endometrioid and clear cell carcinoma of the ovary. Factors affecting survival. Int J Gynecol Pathol. 1989;8(2):132–8.
36. Kim KR, Scully RE. Peritoneal keratin granulomas with carcinomas of endometrium and ovary and atypical polypoid adenomyoma of endometrium. A clinicopathological analysis of 22 cases. Am J Surg Pathol. 1990;14(10):925–32.
37. Katoh T, Yasuda M, Hasegawa K, Kozawa E, Maniwa J, Sasano H. Estrogen-producing endometrioid adenocarcinoma resembling sex cord-stromal tumor of the ovary: a review of four postmenopausal cases. Diagn Pathol. 2012;7:164.
38. Dabbs DJ. Chapter 18: Immunohistology of the female genital tract. In: Diagnostic immunohistochemistory, theranostic and genomic applications. 4th ed. Elsevier Saunders; 2014. p. 683–706.
39. Dabbs DJ, Sturtz K, Zaino RJ. The immunohistochemical discrimination of endometrioid adenocarcinomas. Hum Pathol. 1996;27(2):172–7.
40. Huntsman DG, Clement PB, Gilks CB, Scully RE. Small-cell carcinoma of the endometrium. A clinicopathological study of sixteen cases. Am J Surg Pathol. 1994;18(4):364–75.
41. Houghton O, Connolly LE, McCluggage WG. Morules in endometrioid proliferations of the uterus and ovary consistently express the intestinal transcription factor CDX2. Histopathology. 2008;53(2):156–65.
42. Oliva E, Sarrio D, Brachtel EF, Sanchez-Estevez C, Soslow RA, Moreno-Bueno G, Palacios J. High frequency of beta-catenin mutations in borderline endometrioid tumours of the ovary. J Pathol. 2006;208(5):708–13.
43. Ordi J, Schammel DP, Rasekh L, Tavassoli FA. Sertoliform endometrioid carcinomas of the ovary: a clinicopathologic and immunohistochemical study of 13 cases. Mod Pathol. 1999;12(10):933–40.
44. Misir A, Sur M. Sertoliform endometrioid carcinoma of the ovary: a potential diagnostic pitfall. Arch Pathol Lab Med. 2007;131(6):979–81.
45. Jiang X, Hitchcock A, Bryan EJ, Watson RH, Englefield P, Thomas EJ, Campbell IG. Microsatellite analysis of endometriosis reveals

loss of heterozygosity at candidate ovarian tumor suppressor gene loci. Cancer Res. 1996;56(15):3534–9.
46. Jiang X, Morland SJ, Hitchcock A, Thomas EJ, Campbell IG. Allelotyping of endometriosis with adjacent ovarian carcinoma reveals evidence of a common lineage. Cancer Res. 1998;58(8):1707–12.
47. Obata K, Morland SJ, Watson RH, Hitchcock A, Chenevix-Trench G, Thomas EJ, Campbell IG. Frequent PTEN/MMAC mutations in endometrioid but not serous or mucinous epithelial ovarian tumors. Cancer Res. 1998;58(10):2095–7.
48. Sato N, Tsunoda H, Nishida M, Morishita Y, Takimoto Y, Kubo T, Noguchi M. Loss of heterozygosity on 10q23.3 and mutation of the tumor suppressor gene PTEN in benign endometrial cyst of the ovary: possible sequence progression from benign endometrial cyst to endometrioid carcinoma and clear cell carcinoma of the ovary. Cancer Res. 2000;60(24):7052–6.
49. Madore J, Ren F, Filali-Mouhim A, Sanchez L, Kobel M, Tonin PN, Huntsman D, Provencher DM, Mes-Masson AM. Characterization of the molecular differences between ovarian endometrioid carcinoma and ovarian serous carcinoma. J Pathol. 2010;220(3):392–400.
50. Daly MB. The epidemiology of ovarian cancer. Hematol Oncol Clin North Am. 1992;6(4):729–38.
51. Catasus L, Bussaglia E, Rodrguez I, Gallardo A, Pons C, Irving JA, Prat J. Molecular genetic alterations in endometrioid carcinomas of the ovary: similar frequency of beta-catenin abnormalities but lower rate of microsatellite instability and PTEN alterations than in uterine endometrioid carcinomas. Hum Pathol. 2004;35(11):1360–8.
52. Campbell IG, Russell SE, Choong DY, Montgomery KG, Ciavarella ML, Hooi CS, Cristiano BE, Pearson RB, Phillips WA. Mutation of the PIK3CA gene in ovarian and breast cancer. Cancer Res. 2004;64(21):7678–81.
53. Willner J, Wurz K, Allison KH, Galic V, Garcia RL, Goff BA, Swisher EM. Alternate molecular genetic pathways in ovarian carcinomas of common histological types. Hum Pathol. 2007;38(4):607–13.
54. Wu R, Hendrix-Lucas N, Kuick R, Zhai Y, Schwartz DR, Akyol A, Hanash S, Misek DE, Katabuchi H, Williams BO, Fearon ER, Cho KR. Mouse model of human ovarian endometrioid adenocarcinoma based on somatic defects in the Wnt/beta-catenin and PI3K/Pten signaling pathways. Cancer Cell. 2007;11(4):321–33.
55. Catasus L, Gallardo A, Cuatrecasas M, Prat J. PIK3CA mutations in the kinase domain (exon 20) of uterine endometrial adenocarcinomas are associated with adverse prognostic parameters. Mod Pathol. 2008;21(2):131–9.
56. Gamallo C, Palacios J, Moreno G, Calvo de Mora J, Suarez A, Armas A. Beta-catenin expression pattern in stage I and II ovarian carcinomas : relationship with beta-catenin gene mutations, clinicopathological features, and clinical outcome. Am J Pathol. 1999;155(2):527–36.
57. Moreno-Bueno G, Gamallo C, Perez-Gallego L, Contreras F, Palacios J. Beta-catenin expression in pilomatrixomas. Relationship with beta-catenin gene mutations and comparison with beta-catenin expression in normal hair follicles. Br J Dermatol. 2001;145(4):576–81.
58. Sagae S, Kobayashi K, Nishioka Y, Sugimura M, Ishioka S, Nagata M, Terasawa K, Tokino T, Kudo R. Mutational analysis of beta-catenin gene in Japanese ovarian carcinomas: frequent mutations in endometrioid carcinomas. Jpn J Cancer Res. 1999;90(5):510–5.
59. Wu R, Zhai Y, Fearon ER, Cho KR. Diverse mechanisms of beta-catenin deregulation in ovarian endometrioid adenocarcinomas. Cancer Res. 2001;61(22):8247–55.
60. Wright K, Wilson P, Morland S, Campbell I, Walsh M, Hurst T, Ward B, Cummings M, Chenevix-Trench G. Beta-catenin mutation and expression analysis in ovarian cancer: exon 3 mutations and nuclear translocation in 16% of endometrioid tumours. Int J Cancer. 1999;82(5):625–9.
61. Saegusa M, Okayasu I. Frequent nuclear beta-catenin accumulation and associated mutations in endometrioid-type endometrial and ovarian carcinomas with squamous differentiation. J Pathol. 2001;194(1):59–67.
62. Wiegand KC, Shah SP, Al-Agha OM, Zhao Y, Tse K, Zeng T, Senz J, McConechy MK, Anglesio MS, Kalloger SE, Yang W, Heravi-Moussavi A, Giuliany R, Chow C, Fee J, Zayed A, Prentice L, Melnyk N, Turashvili G, Delaney AD, Madore J, Yip S, McPherson AW, Ha G, Bell L, Fereday S, Tam A, Galletta L, Tonin PN, Provencher D, Miller D, Jones SJ, Moore RA, Morin GB, Oloumi A, Boyd N, Aparicio SA, Shih Ie M, Mes-Masson AM, Bowtell DD, Hirst M, Gilks B, Marra MA, Huntsman DG. ARID1A mutations in endometriosis-associated ovarian carcinomas. N Engl J Med. 2010;363(16):1532–43.
63. Cho KR. Ovarian cancer update: lessons from morphology, molecules, and mice. Arch Pathol Lab Med. 2009;133(11):1775–81.
64. Cho KR, Shih Ie M. Ovarian cancer. Annu Rev Pathol. 2009;4:287–313.
65. McCluggage WG. My approach to and thoughts on the typing of ovarian carcinomas. J Clin Pathol. 2008;61(2):152–63.
66. Schwartz DR, Kardia SL, Shedden KA, Kuick R, Michailidis G, Taylor JM, Misek DE, Wu R, Zhai Y, Darrah DM, Reed H, Ellenson LH, Giordano TJ, Fearon ER, Hanash SM, Cho KR. Gene expression in ovarian cancer reflects both morphology and biological behavior, distinguishing clear cell from other poor-prognosis ovarian carcinomas. Cancer Res. 2002;62(16):4722–9.
67. Cohen PR, Kohn SR, Kurzrock R. Association of sebaceous gland tumors and internal malignancy: the Muir-Torre syndrome. Am J Med. 1991;90(5):606–13.
68. Esche C, Kruse R, Lamberti C, Friedl W, Propping P, Lehmann P, Ruzicka T. Muir-Torre syndrome: clinical features and molecular genetic analysis. Br J Dermatol. 1997;136(6):913–7.
69. Liu J, Albarracin CT, Chang KH, Thompson-Lanza JA, Zheng W, Gershenson DM, Broaddus R, Luthra R. Microsatellite instability and expression of hMLH1 and hMSH2 proteins in ovarian endometrioid cancer. Mod Pathol. 2004;17(1):75–80.
70. Amemiya S, Sekizawa A, Otsuka J, Tachikawa T, Saito H, Okai T. Malignant transformation of endometriosis and genetic alterations of K-ras and microsatellite instability. Int J Gynaecol Obstet. 2004;86(3):371–6.
71. Caduff RF, Svoboda-Newman SM, Bartos RE, Ferguson AW, Frank TS. Comparative analysis of histologic homologues of endometrial and ovarian carcinoma. Am J Surg Pathol. 1998;22(3):319–26.
72. Enomoto T, Weghorst CM, Inoue M, Tanizawa O, Rice JM. K-ras activation occurs frequently in mucinous adenocarcinomas and rarely in other common epithelial tumors of the human ovary. Am J Pathol. 1991;139(4):777–85.
73. Mayr D, Hirschmann A, Lohrs U, Diebold J. KRAS and BRAF mutations in ovarian tumors: a comprehensive study of invasive carcinomas, borderline tumors and extraovarian implants. Gynecol Oncol. 2006;103(3):883–7.
74. Falkenberry SS, Steinhoff MM, Gordinier M, Rappoport S, Gajewski W, Granai CO. Synchronous endometrioid tumors of the ovary and endometrium. A clinicopathologic study of 22 cases. J Reprod Med. 1996;41(10):713–8.
75. Sheu BC, Lin HH, Chen CK, Chao KH, Shun CT, Huang SC. Synchronous primary carcinomas of the endometrium and ovary. Int J Gynaecol Obstet. 1995;51(2):141–6.
76. Soliman PT, Slomovitz BM, Broaddus RR, Sun CC, Oh JC, Eifel PJ, Gershenson DM, Lu KH. Synchronous primary cancers of the endometrium and ovary: a single institution review of 84 cases. Gynecol Oncol. 2004;94(2):456–62.

77. Pearl ML, Johnston CM, Frank TS, Roberts JA. Synchronous dual primary ovarian and endometrial carcinomas. Int J Gynaecol Obstet. 1993;43(3):305–12.
78. Prat J, Matias-Guiu X, Barreto J. Simultaneous carcinoma involving the endometrium and the ovary. A clinicopathologic, immunohistochemical, and DNA flow cytometric study of 18 cases. Cancer. 1991;68(11):2455–9.
79. Bell DA, Scully RE. Benign and borderline clear cell adenofibromas of the ovary. Cancer. 1985;56(12):2922–31.
80. Kao GF, Norris HJ. Unusual cystadenofibromas: endometrioid, mucinous, and clear cell types. Obstet Gynecol. 1979;54(6):729–36.
81. Uzan C, Dufeu-Lefebvre M, Fauvet R, Gouy S, Duvillard P, Darai E, Morice P. Management and prognosis of clear cell borderline ovarian tumor. Int J Gynecol Cancer. 2012;22(6):993–9.
82. Zhao C, Wu LS, Barner R. Pathogenesis of ovarian clear cell adenofibroma, atypical proliferative (borderline) tumor, and carcinoma: clinicopathologic features of tumors with endometriosis or adenofibromatous components support two related pathways of tumor development. J Cancer. 2011;2:94–106.
83. Offman SL, Longacre TA. Clear cell carcinoma of the female genital tract (not everything is as clear as it seems). Adv Anat Pathol. 2012;19(5):296–312.
84. DeLair D, Oliva E, Kobel M, Macias A, Gilks CB, Soslow RA. Morphologic spectrum of immunohistochemically characterized clear cell carcinoma of the ovary: a study of 155 cases. Am J Surg Pathol. 2011;35(1):36–44.
85. Kato N, Takeda J, Fukase M, Motoyama T. Alternate mucoid and hyalinized stroma in clear cell carcinoma of the ovary: manifestation of serial stromal remodeling. Mod Pathol. 2010;23(6):881–8.
86. Clement PB, Young BH. Chapter 14: Surface epithelial–stromal tumors: endometrioid, clear cell, transitional, squamous, rare. In: Atlas of gynecologic surgical pathology. 3rd ed. Elsevier Saunders; 2013.
87. Roth LM, Langley FA, Fox H, Wheeler JE, Czernobilsky B. Ovarian clear cell adenofibromatous tumors. Benign, of low malignant potential, and associated with invasive clear cell carcinoma. Cancer. 1984;53(5):1156–63.
88. Yamamoto S, Tsuda H, Shimazaki H, Takano M, Yoshikawa T, Kuzuya K, Tsuda H, Kurachi H, Kigawa J, Kikuchi Y, Sugiyama T, Matsubara O. Clear cell adenocarcinoma with a component of poorly differentiated histology: a poor prognostic subgroup of ovarian clear cell adenocarcinoma. Int J Gynecol Pathol. 2011;30(5):431–41.
89. Yamamoto S, Tsuda H, Shimazaki H, Takano M, Yoshikawa T, Kuzuya K, Tsuda H, Kurachi H, Kigawa J, Kikuchi Y, Sugiyama T, Matsubara O. Histological grading of ovarian clear cell adenocarcinoma: proposal for a simple and reproducible grouping system based on tumor growth architecture. Int J Gynecol Pathol. 2012;31(2):116–24.
90. Dossus L, Allen N, Kaaks R, Bakken K, Lund E, Tjonneland A, Olsen A, Overvad K, Clavel-Chapelon F, Fournier A, Chabbert-Buffet N, Boeing H, Schutze M, Trichopoulou A, Trichopoulos D, Lagiou P, Palli D, Krogh V, Tumino R, Vineis P, Mattiello A, Bueno-de-Mesquita HB, Onland-Moret NC, Peeters PH, Dumeaux V, Redondo ML, Duell E, Sanchez-Cantalejo E, Arriola L, Chirlaque MD, Ardanaz E, Manjer J, Borgquist S, Lukanova A, Lundin E, Khaw KT, Wareham N, Key T, Chajes V, Rinaldi S, Slimani N, Mouw T, Gallo V, Riboli E. Reproductive risk factors and endometrial cancer: the European Prospective Investigation into Cancer and Nutrition. Int J Cancer. 2010;127(2):442–51.
91. Yamamoto S, Tsuda H, Aida S, Shimazaki H, Tamai S, Matsubara O. Immunohistochemical detection of hepatocyte nuclear factor 1beta in ovarian and endometrial clear-cell adenocarcinomas and nonneoplastic endometrium. Hum Pathol. 2007;38(7):1074–80.
92. Kato N, Sasou S, Motoyama T. Expression of hepatocyte nuclear factor-1beta (HNF-1beta) in clear cell tumors and endometriosis of the ovary. Mod Pathol. 2006;19(1):83–9.
93. Yamashita Y, Nagasaka T, Naiki-Ito A, Sato S, Suzuki S, Toyokuni S, Ito M, Takahashi S. Napsin A is a specific marker for ovarian clear cell adenocarcinoma. Mod Pathol. 2015;28(1):111–7.
94. Alshenawy HA, Radi DA. Napsin-A, a possible diagnostic marker for differentiating clear cell ovarian carcinoma from other high-grade ovarian carcinomas. Appl Immunohistochem Mol Morphol. 2017:1.
95. Nogales FF, Bergeron C, Carvia RE, Alvaro T, Fulwood HR. Ovarian endometrioid tumors with yolk sac tumor component, an unusual form of ovarian neoplasm. Analysis of six cases. Am J Surg Pathol. 1996;20(9):1056–66.
96. Lopez JM, Malpica A, Deavers MT, Ayala AG. Ovarian yolk sac tumor associated with endometrioid carcinoma and mucinous cystadenoma of the ovary. Ann Diagn Pathol. 2003;7(5):300–5.
97. Esheba GE, Pate LL, Longacre TA. Oncofetal protein glypican-3 distinguishes yolk sac tumor from clear cell carcinoma of the ovary. Am J Surg Pathol. 2008;32(4):600–7.
98. Cao D, Guo S, Allan RW, Molberg KH, Peng Y. SALL4 is a novel sensitive and specific marker of ovarian primitive germ cell tumors and is particularly useful in distinguishing yolk sac tumor from clear cell carcinoma. Am J Surg Pathol. 2009;33(6):894–904.
99. Kobel M, Kalloger SE, Carrick J, Huntsman D, Asad H, Oliva E, Ewanowich CA, Soslow RA, Gilks CB. A limited panel of immunomarkers can reliably distinguish between clear cell and high-grade serous carcinoma of the ovary. Am J Surg Pathol. 2009;33(1):14–21.
100. Cameron RI, Ashe P, O'Rourke DM, Foster H, McCluggage WG. A panel of immunohistochemical stains assists in the distinction between ovarian and renal clear cell carcinoma. Int J Gynecol Pathol. 2003;22(3):272–6.
101. Ayhan A, Mao TL, Seckin T, Wu CH, Guan B, Ogawa H, Futagami M, Mizukami H, Yokoyama Y, Kurman RJ, Shih Ie M. Loss of ARID1A expression is an early molecular event in tumor progression from ovarian endometriotic cyst to clear cell and endometrioid carcinoma. Int J Gynecol Cancer. 2012;22(8):1310–5.
102. Jones S, Wang TL, Shih Ie M, Mao TL, Nakayama K, Roden R, Glas R, Slamon D, Diaz LA Jr, Vogelstein B, Kinzler KW, Velculescu VE, Papadopoulos N. Frequent mutations of chromatin remodeling gene ARID1A in ovarian clear cell carcinoma. Science. 2010;330(6001):228–31.
103. Kuo KT, Mao TL, Jones S, Veras E, Ayhan A, Wang TL, Glas R, Slamon D, Velculescu VE, Kuman RJ, Shih Ie M. Frequent activating mutations of PIK3CA in ovarian clear cell carcinoma. Am J Pathol. 2009;174(5):1597–601.
104. Yamamoto S, Tsuda H, Takano M, Iwaya K, Tamai S, Matsubara O. PIK3CA mutation is an early event in the development of endometriosis-associated ovarian clear cell adenocarcinoma. J Pathol. 2011;225(2):189–94.
105. Yamamoto S, Tsuda H, Takano M, Tamai S, Matsubara O. Loss of ARID1A protein expression occurs as an early event in ovarian clear-cell carcinoma development and frequently coexists with PIK3CA mutations. Mod Pathol. 2012;25(4):615–24.
106. Yamamoto S, Tsuda H, Takano M, Hase K, Tamai S, Matsubara O. Clear-cell adenofibroma can be a clonal precursor for clear-cell adenocarcinoma of the ovary: a possible alternative ovarian clear-cell carcinogenic pathway. J Pathol. 2008;216(1):103–10.
107. Cai KQ, Albarracin C, Rosen D, Zhong R, Zheng W, Luthra R, Broaddus R, Liu J. Microsatellite instability and alteration of the expression of hMLH1 and hMSH2 in ovarian clear cell carcinoma. Hum Pathol. 2004;35(5):552–9.
108. Garg K, Leitao MM Jr, Kauff ND, Hansen J, Kosarin K, Shia J, Soslow RA. Selection of endometrial carcinomas for DNA mismatch repair protein immunohistochemistry using patient age and

tumor morphology enhances detection of mismatch repair abnormalities. Am J Surg Pathol. 2009;33(6):925–33.
109. Jensen KC, Mariappan MR, Putcha GV, Husain A, Chun N, Ford JM, Schrijver I, Longacre TA. Microsatellite instability and mismatch repair protein defects in ovarian epithelial neoplasms in patients 50 years of age and younger. Am J Surg Pathol. 2008;32(7):1029–37.
110. Ketabi Z, Bartuma K, Bernstein I, Malander S, Gronberg H, Bjorck E, Holck S, Nilbert M. Ovarian cancer linked to lynch syndrome typically presents as early-onset, non-serous epithelial tumors. Gynecol Oncol. 2011;121(3):462–5.
111. Lu FI, Gilks CB, Mulligan AM, Ryan P, Allo G, Sy K, Shaw PA, Pollett A, Clarke BA. Prevalence of loss of expression of DNA mismatch repair proteins in primary epithelial ovarian tumors. Int J Gynecol Pathol. 2012;31(6):524–31.
112. Hoskins PJ, Le N, Gilks B, Tinker A, Santos J, Wong F, Swenerton KD. Low-stage ovarian clear cell carcinoma: population-based outcomes in British Columbia, Canada, with evidence for a survival benefit as a result of irradiation. J Clin Oncol. 2012;30(14):1656–62.
113. Anglesio MS, Carey MS, Kobel M, Mackay H, Huntsman DG. Clear cell carcinoma of the ovary: a report from the first Ovarian Clear Cell Symposium, June 24th, 2010. Gynecol Oncol. 2011;121(2):407–15.
114. Yamamoto S, Tsuda H, Yoshikawa T, Kudoh K, Kita T, Furuya K, Tamai S, Matsubara O. Clear cell adenocarcinoma associated with clear cell adenofibromatous components: a subgroup of ovarian clear cell adenocarcinoma with distinct clinicopathologic characteristics. Am J Surg Pathol. 2007;31(7):999–1006.
115. Yamamoto S, Tsuda H, Suzuki K, Takano M, Tamai S, Matsubara O. An allelotype analysis indicating the presence of two distinct ovarian clear-cell carcinogenic pathways: endometriosis-associated pathway vs. clear-cell adenofibroma-associated pathway. Virchows Arch. 2009;455(3):261–70.
116. Savvari P, Peitsidis P, Alevizaki M, Dimopoulos MA, Antsaklis A, Papadimitriou CA. Paraneoplastic humorally mediated hypercalcemia induced by parathyroid hormone-related protein in gynecologic malignancies: a systematic review. Onkologie. 2009;32(8–9):517–23.
117. Duska LR, Garrett L, Henretta M, Ferriss JS, Lee L, Horowitz N. When 'never-events' occur despite adherence to clinical guidelines: the case of venous thromboembolism in clear cell cancer of the ovary compared with other epithelial histologic subtypes. Gynecol Oncol. 2010;116(3):374–7.
118. Goff BA, Sainz de la Cuesta R, Muntz HG, Fleischhacker D, Ek M, Rice LW, Nikrui N, Tamimi HK, Cain JM, Greer BE, Fuller AF Jr. Clear cell carcinoma of the ovary: a distinct histologic type with poor prognosis and resistance to platinum-based chemotherapy in stage III disease. Gynecol Oncol. 1996;60(3):412–7.
119. Matsuura Y, Robertson G, Marsden DE, Kim SN, Gebski V, Hacker NF. Thromboembolic complications in patients with clear cell carcinoma of the ovary. Gynecol Oncol. 2007;104(2):406–10.
120. Rahman M, Nakayama K, Rahman MT, Nakayama N, Ishikawa M, Katagiri A, Iida K, Nakayama S, Otsuki Y, Shih Ie M, Miyazaki K. Clinicopathologic and biological analysis of PIK3CA mutation in ovarian clear cell carcinoma. Hum Pathol. 2012;43(12):2197–206.
121. Abe A, Minaguchi T, Ochi H, Onuki M, Okada S, Matsumoto K, Satoh T, Oki A, Yoshikawa H. PIK3CA overexpression is a possible prognostic factor for favorable survival in ovarian clear cell carcinoma. Hum Pathol. 2013;44(2):199–207.
122. Katagiri A, Nakayama K, Rahman MT, Rahman M, Katagiri H, Nakayama N, Ishikawa M, Ishibashi T, Iida K, Kobayashi H, Otsuki Y, Nakayama S, Miyazaki K. Loss of ARID1A expression is related to shorter progression-free survival and chemoresistance in ovarian clear cell carcinoma. Mod Pathol. 2012;25(2):282–8.
123. Rutgers JL, Scully RE. Ovarian mullerian mucinous papillary cystadenomas of borderline malignancy. A clinicopathologic analysis. Cancer. 1988;61(2):340–8.
124. Dube V, Roy M, Plante M, Renaud MC, Tetu B. Mucinous ovarian tumors of Mullerian-type: an analysis of 17 cases including borderline tumors and intraepithelial, microinvasive, and invasive carcinomas. Int J Gynecol Pathol. 2005;24(2):138–46.
125. Rodriguez IM, Irving JA, Prat J. Endocervical-like mucinous borderline tumors of the ovary: a clinicopathologic analysis of 31 cases. Am J Surg Pathol. 2004;28(10):1311–8.
126. Rutgers JL, Scully RE. Ovarian mixed-epithelial papillary cystadenomas of borderline malignancy of mullerian type. A clinicopathologic analysis. Cancer. 1988;61(3):546–54.
127. Shappell HW, Riopel MA, Smith Sehdev AE, Ronnett BM, Kurman RJ. Diagnostic criteria and behavior of ovarian seromucinous (endocervical-type mucinous and mixed cell-type) tumors: atypical proliferative (borderline) tumors, intraepithelial, microinvasive, and invasive carcinomas. Am J Surg Pathol. 2002;26(12):1529–41.
128. Wu CH, Mao TL, Vang R, Ayhan A, Wang TL, Kurman RJ, Shih Ie M. Endocervical-type mucinous borderline tumors are related to endometrioid tumors based on mutation and loss of expression of ARID1A. Int J Gynecol Pathol. 2012;31(4):297–303.
129. Seidman JD, Soslow RA, Vang R, Berman JJ, Stoler MH, Sherman ME, Oliva E, Kajdacsy-Balla A, Berman DM, Copeland LJ. Borderline ovarian tumors: diverse contemporary viewpoints on terminology and diagnostic criteria with illustrative images. Hum Pathol. 2004;35(8):918–33.
130. Nagai Y, Kishimoto T, Nikaido T, Nishihara K, Matsumoto T, Suzuki C, Ogishima T, Kuwahara Y, Hurukata Y, Mizunuma M, Nakata Y, Ishikura H. Squamous predominance in mixed-epithelial papillary cystadenomas of borderline malignancy of mullerian type arising in endometriotic cysts: a study of four cases. Am J Surg Pathol. 2003;27(2):242–7.
131. Lin X, Lindner JL, Silverman JF, Liu Y. Intestinal type and endocervical-like ovarian mucinous neoplasms are immunophenotypically distinct entities. Appl Immunohistochem Mol Morphol. 2008;16(5):453–8.
132. Vang R, Gown AM, Barry TS, Wheeler DT, Ronnett BM. Ovarian atypical proliferative (borderline) mucinous tumors: gastrointestinal and seromucinous (endocervical-like) types are immunophenotypically distinctive. Int J Gynecol Pathol. 2006;25(1):83–9.
133. Yasunaga M, Ohishi Y, Oda Y, Misumi M, Iwasa A, Kurihara S, Nishimura I, Okuma E, Kobayashi H, Wake N, Tsuneyoshi M. Immunohistochemical characterization of mullerian mucinous borderline tumors: possible histogenetic link with serous borderline tumors and low-grade endometrioid tumors. Hum Pathol. 2009;40(7):965–74.
134. Lee KR, Nucci MR. Ovarian mucinous and mixed epithelial carcinomas of mullerian (endocervical-like) type: a clinicopathologic analysis of four cases of an uncommon variant associated with endometriosis. Int J Gynecol Pathol. 2003;22(1):42–51.
135. Taylor J, McCluggage WG. Ovarian seromucinous carcinoma: report of a series of a newly categorized and uncommon neoplasm. Am J Surg Pathol. 2015;39(7):983–92.
136. Rambau PF, McIntyre JB, Taylor J, Lee S, Ogilvie T, Sienko A, Morris D, Duggan MA, McCluggage WG, Kobel M. Morphologic reproducibility, genotyping, and immunohistochemical profiling do not support a category of seromucinous carcinoma of the ovary. Am J Surg Pathol. 2017;41(5):685–95.

6 Problems with the Histological Diagnosis of Epithelial Borderline Tumors of the Ovary

Miki Kushima

Abstract

The pathological diagnosis of epithelial borderline tumors (serous, mucinous, endometrioid, Brenner, and seromucinous) of the ovary can be difficult due to some problems in the gynecological pathology: (1) conflicting definitions of epithelial borderline tumor, in particular, when it is difficult to determine the degree of nuclear atypia and microinvasion of the serous borderline tumor, (2) distinction between primary and metastatic mucinous tumor, (3) difficulties in the intraoperative diagnosis of mucinous tumors, (4) difference between squamous metaplasia and solid growth of epithelial tumor cells in endometrioid tumor, (5) difficulty and rarity of the diagnosis of clear cell borderline tumor and borderline Brenner tumor, and (6) diagnosis of seromucinous borderline tumor.

The nuclear grade and the absence of obvious stromal invasion are principal diagnostic criterions for borderline tumors. The intracystic exophytic papillary proliferations are a typical finding of the borderline tumor. However, there are problems with predominantly tubular and cystic tumors, such as those of mucinous, endometrioid, and clear cell types. The definition of microinvasion is that up to 5 mm in maximum dimension. Borderline tumors with stromal microinvasion should be distinguished from small foci of (microinvasive) carcinoma arising in a borderline tumor.

Keywords

Ovary · Epithelial borderline tumor · Histological diagnosis

Epithelial borderline (atypical proliferative) ovarian tumors were first recognized as a distinct category by Taylor in 1929 who used terminologies like "semi-malignant" and "borderline" to describe them [1]. In 1961 the Cancer Committee of the International Federation of Gynecology and Obstetrics (FIGO) proposed a histopathological classification of the common epithelial ovarian tumors. As a part of this classification, a new category was introduced that was designated "serous cystadenomas with proliferating activity of the epithelial cells and nuclear abnormalities but with no infiltrative destructive growth (low potential malignancy)" [2]. The FIGO classification was accepted by WHO and published in 1973, but the above term was changed to "tumors of borderline malignancy (carcinomas of low malignant potential)." And this term evolved into "borderline malignancy," which has been widely used, the implication being that this group of tumors had morphological features and behavior between a benign cystadenoma and carcinoma. Subsequent WHO classifications (2014) separated this group from carcinomas and termed them as atypical proliferative ovarian tumors or borderline tumors [2].

The pathological diagnosis of epithelial borderline tumors of the ovary can be difficult due to some problems in the gynecological pathology. The problems in histological diagnosis of epithelial borderline tumors are as follows: (1) conflicting definitions of epithelial borderline tumor, in particular, when it is difficult to determine the degree of nuclear atypia and microinvasion of the serous borderline tumor, (2) distinction between primary and metastatic mucinous tumor, (3) difficulties in the intraoperative diagnosis of mucinous tumors, (4) difference between squamous metaplasia and solid growth of epithelial tumor cells in endometrioid tumor, (5) difficulty and rarity of the diagnosis of clear cell borderline tumor and borderline Brenner tumor, and (6) diagnosis of seromucinous borderline tumor. In the following sections, the basis for these problems will be described.

M. Kushima
Department of Pathology, Showa University, School of Medicine, Showa University Koto Toyosu Hospital, Tokyo, Japan
e-mail: mkushima@med.showa-u.ac.jp

T. Moriya (ed.), *Pathology of Female Cancers*, https://doi.org/10.1007/978-981-10-8606-9_6

6.1 Serous Tumor

Benign serous tumors consist of epithelial cells resembling those of the fallopian tube, including ciliated cells. There are three types of tumor morphology: cystadenoma, adenofibroma, and surface papilloma. When <10% of the epithelial volume shows epithelial stratification and cellular atypia like SBT (serous borderline tumor)/APST (atypical proliferative serous tumor), such tumors are designated serous cystadenoma/adenofibroma with focal epithelial proliferation. Serous borderline tumor (SBP) and low-grade serous carcinoma (LGSC) are part of one biological continuum, whereby SBP can transform into LGSC. It has been suggested that some nodal SBPs arise from nodal endosalpingiosis and evolve independently in lymph nodes (rather than being related to the primary ovarian carcinoma) [3].

Serous borderline tumors/atypical proliferative serous tumors (SBTs/APSTs) are defined as noninvasive tumors with greater epithelial proliferation and cytologic atypia (Figs. 6.1, 6.2 and 6.3), rather than benign serous tumor with less than low-grade serous carcinoma [2]. However, the behavior of ovarian serous borderline tumors and the significance of various prognostic factors remain unclear, and they are difficult to evaluate because of the inconsistencies and disagreement in the literature [4].

The pathological diagnosis of serous borderline tumors presents the following problems:

1. The first problem is difficulty of diagnosis regarding the degree of nuclear atypia.
2. The second problem is the definition of microinvasion (Fig. 6.4) and the presence of implants in the peritoneum.
3. The third problem is endosalpingiosis and clusters of eosinophilic epithelial-type cells in the pelvic lymph nodes.
4. The final problem is the serous borderline tumor-micropapillary variant which has less nuclear atypia than the common serous borderline tumor, but it presents with more advanced-stage disease.

Serous borderline tumors have papillary and tubular structures, which consist of epithelial tumor cells with mild to moderate nuclear atypia, round and ovoid nuclei without marked enlarged nucleoli, and severe atypia, such as that seen in high-grade serous carcinoma.

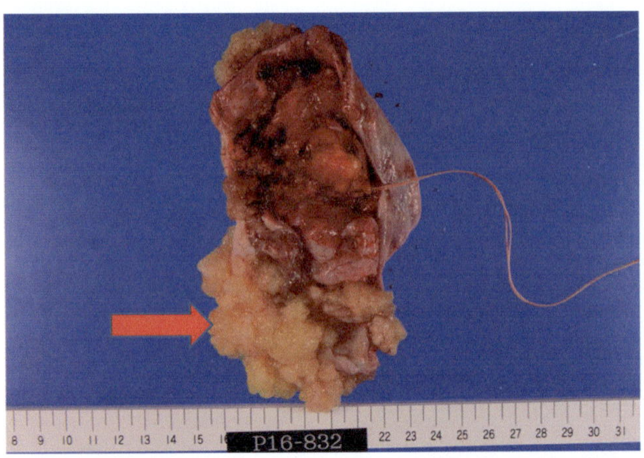

Fig. 6.1 Macroscopic findings of the cut surface of a serous borderline tumor. There are many papillary structures (arrow) in the large cystic lesion

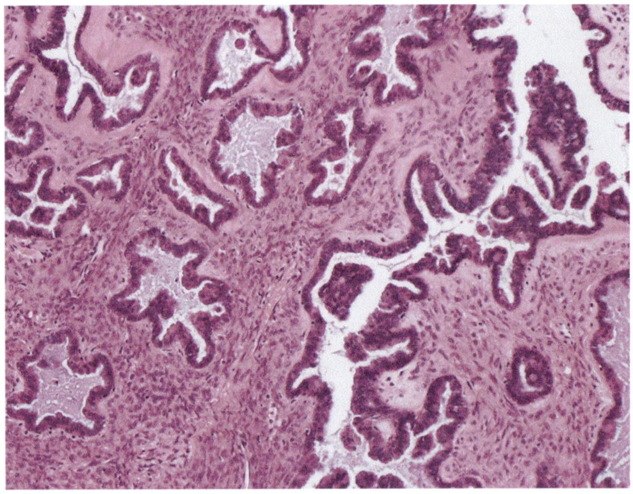

Fig. 6.2 Serous borderline tumor/atypical proliferative serous tumor (SBT/APST). Hierarchical and branching architecture lined by cuboidal and columnar epithelia

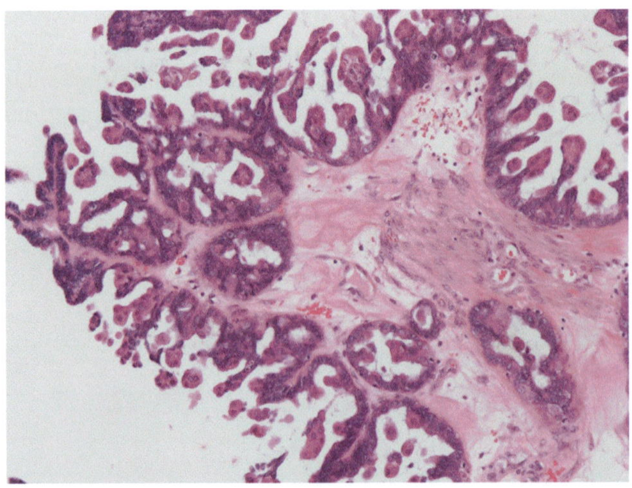

Fig. 6.3 Serous borderline tumor/atypical proliferative serous tumor. Papillary proliferation of eosinophilic cells, which are detached clusters floating above the papillae, is seen

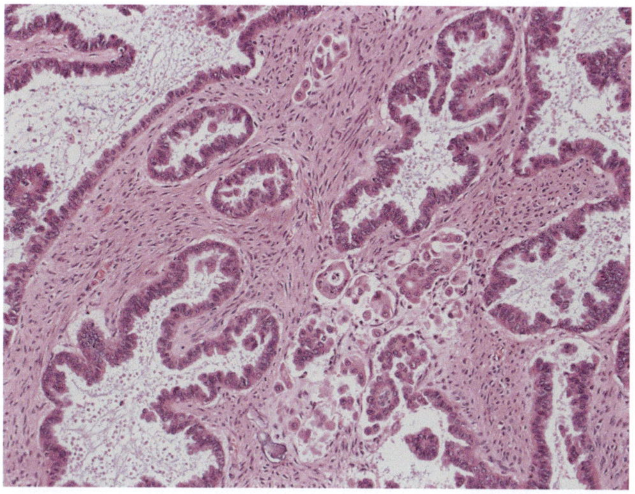

Fig. 6.4 Small focus of microinvasion in a serous borderline tumor. Some clusters of cells in the stroma have abundant eosinophilic cytoplasm

Microinvasion in the primary ovarian tumor was associated with a 100% survival rate at 6.7 years. Figure 6.3 shows microinvasion of the serous borderline tumor with single to small clusters of atypical epithelial cells with eosinophilic cytoplasm in the stroma. The lesion is <5 mm at the greatest dimension. When there are multiple small groups of carcinomatous cells, this is not considered as microinvasion, but rather "microinvasive carcinoma."

Noninvasive implants are confined to the surface of the organs, but the most reliable prognostic indicator for advanced-stage tumors is peritoneal invasive implants.

Lymph node involvement (LNI) was associated with a 98% survival rate at 6.5 years [4]. There was no significant difference in survival for patients with LNI compared with patients without LNI. However, the presence of discrete nodular aggregates of the epithelium of greater than 1 mm in linear dimension, with no intervening lymphoid tissue, was associated with a statistically significant decreased disease-free survival when compared with other patterns of LNI ($P = 0.02$) [5]. It has been suggested that some nodal serous borderline tumors arise from nodal endosalpingiosis and evolve independently in lymph nodes (rather than being related to the primary ovarian carcinoma) [3].

Serous borderline tumor-micropapillary variant/noninvasive low-grade serous carcinoma is a noninvasive ovarian tumor with a micropapillary and non-hierarchical branching architecture with micropapillary and/or cribriform patterns composed of rounded cells. The tumor cells have scant cytoplasm and moderate nuclear atypia [2]. Both the serous borderline tumor and low-grade serous carcinoma are characterized by occasional mutations of the KRAS or BRAF genes and the lack of TP53 gene mutation [6].

Interestingly, however, there is differential gene expression between this tumor (low-grade noninvasive serous carcinoma) and the former tumor (serous borderline tumor) based on gene expression profile studies (WHO textbook 2014) [2]. Further, the expression between noninvasive low-grade serous carcinoma and invasive low-grade serous carcinoma does not differ.

The nuclear grade is the most important diagnostic feature in the differentiation between low-grade serous carcinoma and high-grade serous carcinoma [6].

6.1.1 Molecular Studies in Ovarian Serous Borderline Tumors (SBTs)

In SBTs, Kras mutations range from 17 to 39.5%, while Braf mutations range from 23 to 48% [7]. Kras and Braf mutations represent very early events in the tumorigenesis of SBT as both are detected in serous cystadenomas associated with SBTs [7]. Serous cystadenomas seem to progress to SBT as a result of a Braf mutation, but this mutation is rarely involved in the progression to low-grade serous carcinoma (LGSC). SBTs with a Braf mutation are associated with cellular senescence and upregulation of tumor suppressor genes.

6.2 Mucinous Tumor

The incidence of ovarian mucinous tumor is relatively higher in Japan [8] than in Western countries.

The following four problems complicate the pathological diagnosis of mucinous tumor of the ovary [8]:

1. Conflicting definitions of borderline tumors. In particular, the so-called endocervical-like-type mucinous borderline tumor, which is composed of broad bulbous papillae and intracystic growth, looks like those in serous borderline tumors and has been considered a subset of mucinous tumors in the past. These tumors are considered seromucinous borderline tumors according to the WHO classification (2014).
2. Mural nodules within mucinous cystic tumors are malignant (anaplastic carcinoma, sarcoma, and carcinosarcoma) or benign (sarcoma-like).
3. Differential diagnosis in primary vs. metastatic mucinous tumors from other organs including the appendix, colon, stomach, pancreas, or uterine cervix. These tumors have histological findings similar to those of primary ovarian mucinous tumors (benign, borderline, and malignant).
4. Difficulties in the intraoperative rapid diagnosis of mucinous ovarian tumors [8].

Mucinous borderline tumor/atypical proliferating mucinous tumor are composed of mild to moderate atypical gastrointestinal-type mucin-containing epithelial cells either without invasion or with a small stromal invasion measuring less than 5 mm in the greatest linear extent [2]. The presence of minimal stratification and slight nuclear atypia does not define a mucinous borderline tumor. Mucinous borderline tumors show evident stratification, tufting, and papillary structure of the epithelial tumor cells with mild to moderate atypia (Fig. 6.5). High-grade nuclear atypia is confined to the epithelium in mucinous intraepithelial carcinoma. This tumor is diagnosed based on the precise observation of the histologic specimen. The important points of mucinous borderline tumors are as follows: (1) Small areas of extravasation of the mucin and mucinous granulomas are present in benign and mucinous borderline tumors (Fig. 6.6). (2) Tumor heterogeneity is common in mucinous tumors, such that it may include benign and/or borderline components in the same and/or different areas of a single tumor [8].

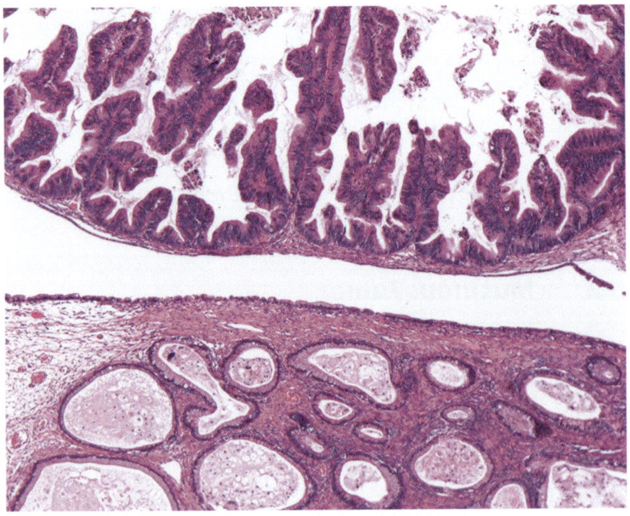

Fig. 6.5 Mucinous borderline tumor component (upper) and benign mucinous adenofibroma-like lesion (lower) in the same tumor

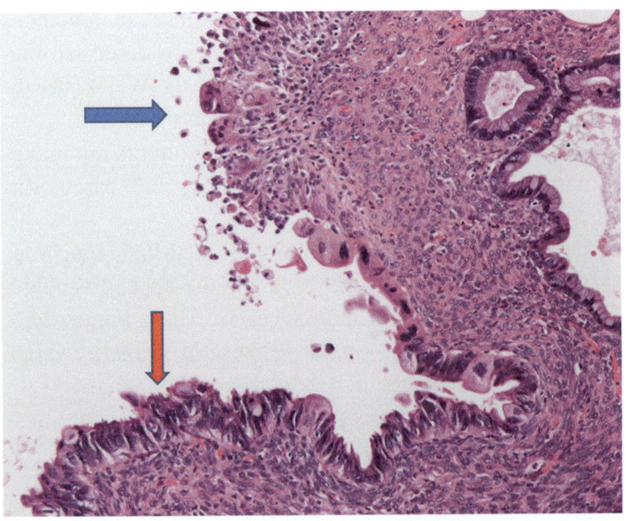

Fig. 6.6 Mucinous borderline tumor with intraepithelial carcinoma-like lesion (red arrow) and mucinous granuloma (blue arrow)

Adequate sampling of the mucinous borderline tumor is important. Sampling of these tumors must include up to one histologic section per 1–2 cm tumor diameter as well as the sampling of any suspicious lesions, such as multilocular and solid areas including mural nodules.

It is the differential diagnosis between primary and metastatic mucinous tumors that is the critical point for therapy. Primary mucinous borderline tumors arise from mucinous cystadenoma, teratoma, and Brenner tumors. Metastatic mucinous tumors are from the appendix, large intestine, stomach, pancreas, and uterine cervix. These tumors have histological findings similar to those of primary mucinous ovarian tumors, (benign, borderline, and malignant). Immunohistochemical staining of CK7 is diffusely positive, and CK20 is negative to less extensive compared to CK7; 50–60% of tumors are positive for PAX8 [2].

The mural nodule can be associated with mucinous borderline tumor, reactive sarcoma-like mural nodules, foci of anaplastic carcinoma, and sarcomatous nodules. In some cases, anaplastic carcinomatous mural nodules in ovarian mucinous tumors display the same *K-RAS* mutation as their underlying neoplasm. This finding provides supportive evidence that at least some malignant mural nodules represent a form of dedifferentiation in ovarian mucinous tumor [9].

In intraoperative rapid diagnosis, a false-negative diagnosis from frozen sections can occur due to limited sampling, as in clinical practice only a few frozen sections (1 or 2) can be taken from each tumor. And cytological specimens (scrape or imprint smears) which are sampled from any suspicious lesions or from almost all cut surfaces of the tumors can facilitate rapid diagnosis of mucinous ovarian tumor [8].

6.3 Endometrioid Tumor

Endometrioid tumors may develop within the endometriotic cyst and endometriosis. Benign endometrioid tumors include the following: endometriotic cyst, endometrioid cystadenoma, and adenofibroma. Endometrioid carcinoma is the second most common malignant tumor of the ovary; however, atypical proliferative endometrioid ovarian tumor or borderline endometrioid ovarian tumor constitutes a minuscule 0.2% among all ovarian surface epithelial tumors [10].

Endometrioid borderline tumor/atypical proliferative tumor is a solid or cystic tumor with epithelial proliferation, mild to moderate cytological atypia, epithelial stratification, and squamous (morular) metaplasia (Figs. 6.7 and 6.8). These tumors are composed of crowded glands and may show back-to-back proliferation with fibrous stroma (adenofibromatous) or a papillary growth pattern which protrudes into cystic structures (intracystic). Endometrioid borderline tumor is uncommon (0.2% of the epithelial ovarian tumor) [2]. Many endometrioid borderline tumors have associated endometriosis of the ovary and coexisting endometrial hyperplasia and/or endometrial carcinoma of the uterus.

Atypical proliferative (borderline) endometrioid tumors (APTs) and well-differentiated endometrioid carcinomas of the ovary constitute a spectrum of morphologically diverse proliferative tumors. There is currently no agreement on the criteria for distinguishing between the two types [11]. Microinvasion has been defined in two ways: (1) confluent glandular growth <5 mm or (2) haphazard infiltrating single cells, glands, or nests of cells with cytologic atypia. In particular, the borderline tumors, which have confluent glandular growth <5 mm with cytologic atypia and squamous metaplasia (morula), should not be mistaken for invasive carcinoma.

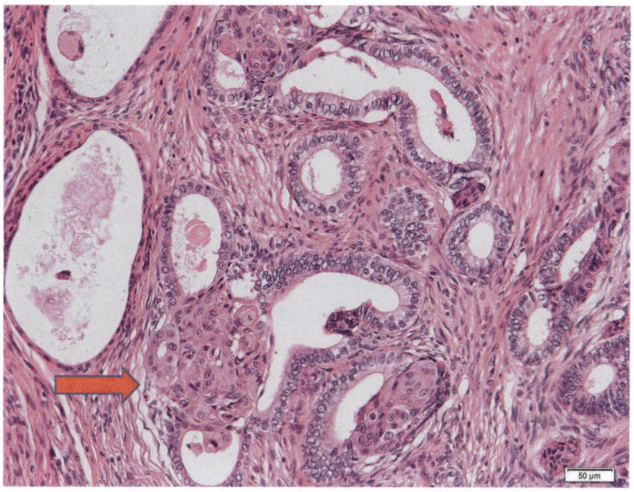

Fig. 6.7 Endometrioid tumor with morula (red arrow) and fibrous stroma (adenofibroma)

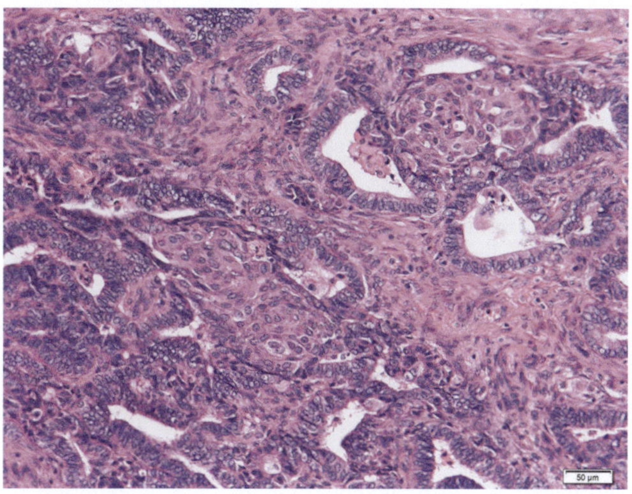

Fig. 6.8 Another case of endometrioid borderline tumor with more complex structures. There is no stromal invasion

As for the background, half of the cases of borderline tumors are adenofibroma. Mild to moderate cytological atypia with stratification (EIN/atypical hyperplasia-like) is seen in endometrioid borderline tumors. The epithelial proliferation may result in bridging and a cribriform growth pattern. Squamous (morular) metaplasia and complex glandular structure (fusion of glands or small focus of cribriform pattern) of the epithelium should not be mistaken for invasive carcinoma.

6.4 Clear Cell Tumors

Clear cell tumors of the ovary are relatively uncommon; most are clear cell carcinomas. Benign and borderline clear cell tumors are extremely rare and when seen, they are almost always fibromatous [12].

Clear cell borderline tumor/atypical proliferative clear cell tumor is a clear cell adenofibromous or a cystadenomatous tumor with mild to moderate atypia without stromal invasion. Both types of clear cell tumors, adenofibromatous and cystic, appear to be derived from endometriosis. However, the former type develops from non-cystic endometriosis, and it is associated with adenofibromatous components, while the latter type arises from an endometriotic cyst (endometrioma) and is not associated with an adenofibromatous background [13]. The tumor is histologically composed of a tubular component lined in part with flat or cuboidal clear, as well as hobnail cells with clear or eosinophilic cytoplasm. The tumor cells have mild cytologic atypia and abundant stromal components. Figure 6.9 shows a large cyst wall and a nodular adenofibromatous lesion. Dilated glands consist of single to slightly stratified epithelial cells with clear

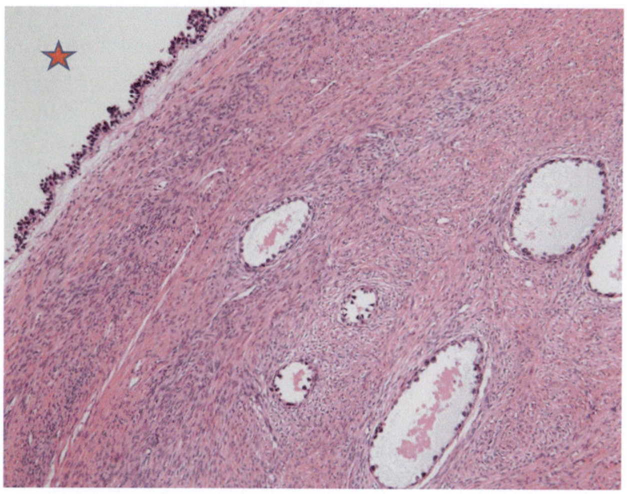

Fig. 6.9 Clear cell tumor with a large cyst (star) and a nodular adenofibromatous lesions. Dilated glands which consist of single to slightly stratified epithelial cells with clear and eosinophilic cytoplasm in the nodular lesions. Some epithelial cells show mild atypia

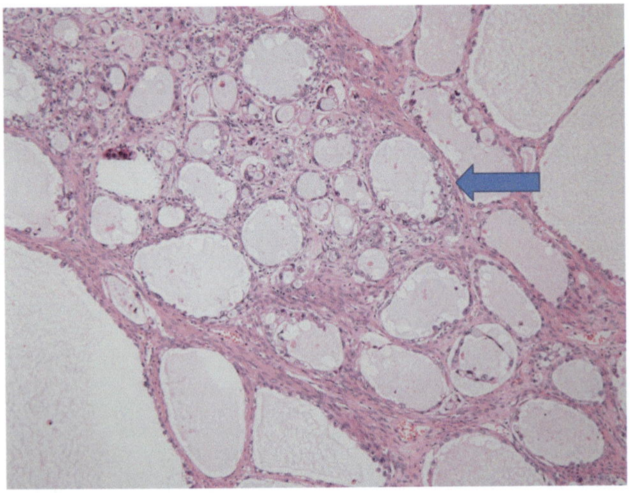

Fig. 6.10 Clear cell tumor with microinvasion (arrow)

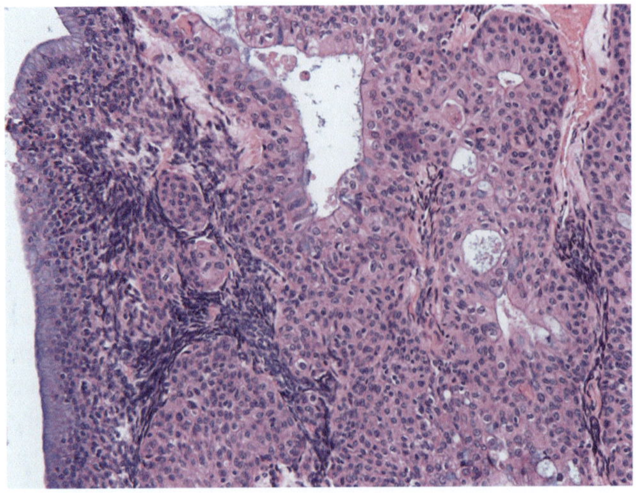

Fig. 6.11 Brenner tumor with atypical proliferation. This finding looks like transitional (urothelial) epithelium

and eosinophilic cytoplasm in the nodular lesions. Some epithelial cells show mild atypia.

Figure 6.10 shows a small focus of stromal invasion (invasive clear cell carcinoma) in a clear cell borderline tumor (adenofibromatous lesion). This tumor was diagnosed as clear cell carcinoma, based on the clearly abnormal architecture indicative of invasion.

The epithelial cells of clear cell borderline tumors have diastase-digestive PAS-positive material in the cytoplasm, and occasionally the luminal surface and intraluminal substance are stained with mucicarmine. Some of the epithelial cells show positive lipid staining with Sudan III stain. On ultrastructural study, the tumors feature a moderate number of small mitochondria, poorly developed rough endoplasmic reticulum (rER), short microvilli, intercellular tight junction and desmosome, and a few glycogen granules [14].

Recently, Skirnisdottir et al. (2013) [15] and Yamashita et al. (2015) [16] proposed that napsin A is a sensitive and specific marker to differentiate ovarian clear cell tumors (especially adenocarcinomas) from other ovarian tumors. Yamashita et al. reported that in 71 of 86 ovarian clear cell adenocarcinoma patients (83%) and in all 13 ovarian clear cell adenofibroma patients, positive napsin A staining was evident by immunohistochemical analysis.

6.5 Brenner Tumors

From the WHO classification, Brenner tumors present the following forms: benign, borderline, and malignant. The benign tumors are the most frequent and account for approximately 95%. Histologically, benign Brenner tumors consist of characteristic oval or irregular nests of transitional-type cells with longitudinal grooves in the nuclei of the tumor cells. The borderline Brenner tumors represent about 5% and the malignant tumors less than 1%.

Borderline Brenner tumor/atypical proliferative Brenner tumor shows a transitional cell type of epithelial proliferation of crowded nests (Fig. 6.11). Borderline Brenner tumors represent quite a rare entity of ovarian tumors (about 2%). They are formed from papillary structures made of fibrovascular conjunctive axes covered by a transition epithelium, which is similar to that of the urinary bladder epithelium [17]. The histogenesis of the benign Brenner tumor is not well characterized, but borderline Brenner tumors are suspected to arise from benign tumors.

To date, about 30 cases of Brenner borderline tumors have been described in accordance with the WHO classification; all were characterized by the absence of stromal infiltration and the association with a benign component [18]. These lesions seem to originate from transitional metaplasia of the tubal epithelial cells [18]. Tumor cells show mild to moderate nuclear atypia. Stromal invasion is absent. Mucinous metaplasia is often present [2].

Immunohistochemical stains for p63 and GATA3 are usually positive [2]. Borderline Brenner tumors are negative for WT-1, p16, Rb, and p53 and show weak immunostaining for cyclin D1, moderate for Ras, and strong for EGFR [18].

6.6 Seromucinous Tumors

The recent 2014 World Health Organization (WHO) Classification of Tumours of the Female Reproductive Organs [2] introduced a new category of ovarian neoplasm designated as "seromucinous tumors." The recognition of this distinctive group of tumors is an important addition to the classification [19].

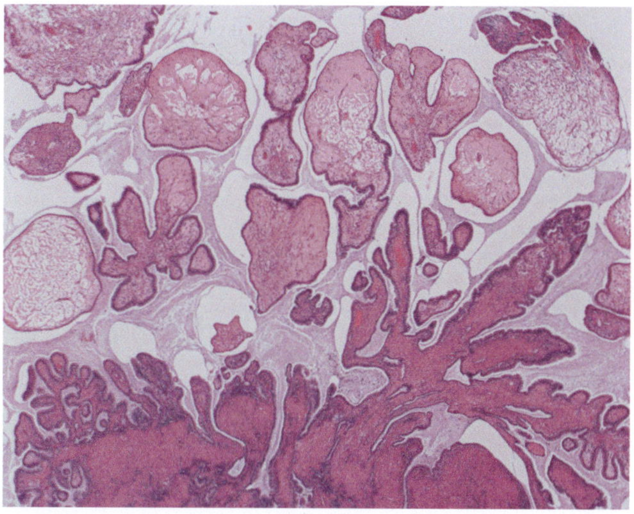

Fig. 6.12 Seromucinous borderline tumor. Papillary proliferative structures

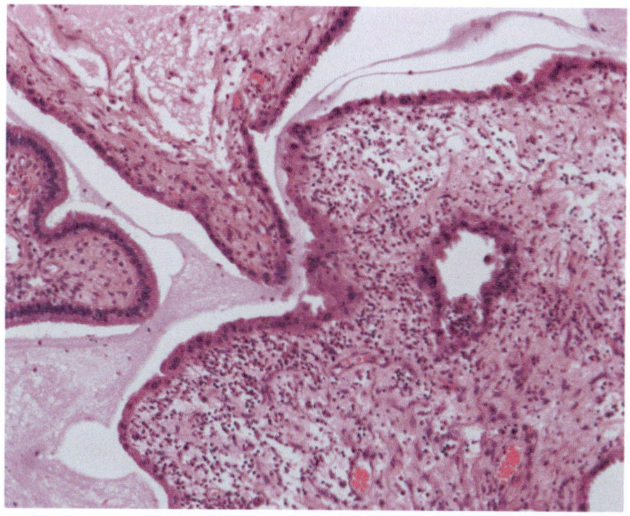

Fig. 6.13 Seromucinous borderline tumor with inflammatory cellular infiltration in the stroma

These tumors often contain endocervical-type mucinous epithelium, but they typically display a papillary architecture, unlike most endocervical neoplasms, and their immunophenotype is different from both endocervical and serous tumors. Moreover, they frequently contain ciliated cells, endometrial-type cells, cells with abundant eosinophilic cytoplasm, and hobnail-shaped cells, all of which can be found in endometrioid tumors [20].

However, the term "seromucinous" is controversial. Kurman and Shih [19] suggested that, based on the clinicopathologic, immunohistochemical and molecular genetic features, a more appropriate designation for this group of tumors is "mixed Mullerian tumors" which can be subcategorized as "mixed Mullerian cystadenomas," "mixed Mullerian atypical proliferative (borderline) tumors," and "mixed Mullerian carcinomas."

Seromucinous borderline tumor (SMBT)/atypical proliferative seromucinous tumor is a noninvasive proliferative epithelial tumor composed of mixed cell type, most often serous, and endocervical-like type. Endometrioid, clear cell [21] transitional, and squamous cells are also seen in the same tumor. Ovarian seromucinous borderline tumors, although characterized by papillary architecture reminiscent of serous tumors (Fig. 6.12), are composed of mucinous epithelium similar to that of the endocervix. The neutrophilic infiltration is seen in the stroma of the papillae (Fig. 6.13). These tumors are often associated with endometriosis.

ARID1A is a tumor suppressor, which frequently loses its expression and is mutated in endometrium-related carcinomas, including ovarian clear cell, ovarian endometrioid, and uterine endometrioid carcinomas. Loss of ARID1A staining was shown in 8 (33%) of 24 seromucinous tumors. In contrast, ARID1A staining was retained in all 32 tumors, except for 1 endometrioid tumor ($P < 0.01$) [20]. Endometriosis-related ovarian neoplasms (ERONs) are a unique group of tumors as they are associated with endometriosis and, in particular, endometriosis presenting as an ovarian endometriotic cyst (endometrioma). ERONs include clear cell carcinoma, endometrioid carcinoma, and seromucinous borderline tumor [22].

The differentiation of SMBT from endometriosis-related malignant ovarian tumor is clinically important. In MR imaging findings, the following quantitative values were evaluated using receiver-operating characteristic analysis: overall and solid portion sizes, fluid signal intensity (SI), degree of contrast enhancement, and mean and minimum apparent diffusion coefficient (ADC) values of the solid portion. The diagnostic performance of quantitative values of mean and minimum apparent diffusion coefficient (ADC) values of the solid portion was the most useful value. "T2WI high SI solid portion" was the most useful MRI finding [23].

Conclusions

Epithelial borderline tumor seems to be a popular topic among gynecologic pathologists and gynecologists. "Atypical proliferating (or atypical proliferative) tumor" is the synonym of borderline tumor in the recently published 2014 WHO classification. However, to date the concept and terminology for borderline tumors continues to be problematic at the present time.

The nuclear grade and the absence of obvious stromal invasion are principal diagnostic criterions for borderline tumors. The intracystic exophytic papillary proliferations are a typical finding of the borderline tumor. However, there are problems with predominantly tubular and cystic tumors, such as those of mucinous, endometrioid, and clear cell types. The latter has a fused and cribriform pattern of glands and cysts with minimal stromal components and stromal desmoplastic reaction. The definition of microinvasion is that up to 5 mm in maximum dimension. However, some investigators have pointed out that the maximum size has not been scientifically validated nor has the number of allowable foci. Borderline tumors with stromal microinvasion should be distinguished from small foci of (microinvasive) carcinoma arising in a borderline tumor.

In intraoperative rapid diagnosis of mucinous tumor, a false-negative diagnosis from frozen sections can occur due to limited sampling. It is important that we comprehend the limitations of the frozen section in intraoperative rapid diagnosis. And the cytological specimens (scrape or imprint smears), which are sampled from suspicious lesions or from almost all cut surfaces of the tumors, can facilitate rapid diagnosis of various types of ovarian tumors [8], including borderline epithelial tumors.

Acknowledgments I would like to express my sincere appreciation to the staffs of the Department of Pathology, Showa University Hospital, Fujigaoka Hospital and Koto Toyosu Hospital for long-standing supports.

References

1. Taylor H. Malignant and semi-malignant tumors of the ovary. Surg Gynecol Obstet. 1929;48:204–30.
2. Kurman RJ, Carcangiu ML, Herrington CS, Young RH, editors. WHO Classification of tumors of female reproductive organs. Chapter 1. Tumor of the ovary. Lyon: IARC; 2014. p. 18–20.
3. Djordjevic B, Malpica A. Ovarian serous tumors of low malignant potential with nodal low-grade serous carcinoma. Am J Surg Pathol. 2012;36(7):955–63.
4. Seidman JD, Kurman RJ. Ovarian serous borderline tumors: a critical review of the literature with emphasis on prognostic indicators. Hum Pathol. 2000;31(5):539–57.
5. JK MK, Balzer BL, Longacre TA. Lymph node involvement in ovarian serous tumors of low malignant potential (borderline tumors): pathology, prognosis, and proposed classification. Am J Surg Pathol. 2006;30(5):614–24.
6. Ohishi Y, Imamura H, Aman M, Shida K, Kaku T, Kato K, Oda Y. Is invasive micropapillary serous carcinoma a low-grade carcinoma? Int J Gynecol Pathol. 2015;35(1):56–65.
7. Malpica A, Wong KK. The molecular pathology of ovarian serous borderline tumors. Ann Oncol. 2016;27(Suppl 1):i16–9. https://doi.org/10.1093/annonc/mdw089.
8. Kushima M. Problems in the pathological diagnosis and intraoperative rapid diagnosis of mucinous tumor of the ovary. Showa Univ J Med Sci. 2013;25(1):1–7.
9. Desouki MM, Dineo Khabele D, Crispens MA, Fadare O. Ovarian mucinous tumor with malignant mural nodules: Dedifferentiation or collision? Int J Gynecol Pathol. 2015;34(1):19–24.
10. Roth LM, Emerson RE, Ulbright TM. Ovarian endometrioid tumors of low malignant potential: A clinicopathologic study of 30 cases with comparison to well-differentiated endometrioid adenocarcinoma. Am J Surg Pathol. 2003;27:1253–9.
11. Bell KA, Kurman RJ. A clinicopathologic analysis of atypical proliferative (borderline) tumors and well-differentiated endometrioid adenocarcinomas of the ovary. Am J Surg Pathol. 2000;24(11):1465–79.
12. Vasilakaki T, Skafida E, Arkoumani E, Grammatoglou X, Firfiris N, Manoloudaki K. Borderline clear cell adenofibroma of the ovary associated with ovarian endometriosis: a case report. Eur J Gynaecol Oncol. 2012;33(2):230–2.
13. Zhao C, Wu LS, Barner R. Pathogenesis of ovarian clear cell adenofibroma, atypical proliferative (borderline) tumor, and carcinoma: clinicopathologic features of tumors with endometriosis or adenofibromatous components support two related pathways of tumor development. J Cancer. 2011;2:94–106. https://doi.org/10.7150/jca.2.94.
14. Katsube Y, Fujiwara H, Tanioka Y, Imajo M, Fujiwara A. Ovarian clear cell adenofibroma of borderline malignancy. A case report. Hiroshima J Med Sci. 1989;38(2):87–90.
15. Skirnisdottir I, Bjersand K, Åkerud H, Seidal T. Napsin A as a marker of clear cell ovarian carcinoma. BMC Cancer. 2013;13:524. https://doi.org/10.1186/1471-2407-13-524.
16. Yamashita Y, Nagasaka T, Naiki-Ito A, Sato S, Suzuki S, Toyokuni S, Ito M, Takahashi S. Napsin A is a specific marker for ovarian clear cell adenocarcinoma. Mod Pathol. 2015;28:111–7.
17. Albu DF, Albu CC, Gogănău AM, Albu ŞD, Mogoantă L, Edu A, DiTescu D, Văduva CC. Borderline Brenner tumors associated with ovarian cyst - case presentation. Rom J Morphol Embryol. 2016;57(2 Suppl):893–8.
18. Cecio RD, Cantile M, Collina F, Marra L, Santonastaso C, Scaffa C, Botti G, Losito NS. Borderline Brenner tumor of the ovary: a case report with immunohistochemical and molecular study. J Ovarian Res. 2014;**7**:101.
19. Kurman RJ, Shih IM. Seromucinous tumors of the ovary. What's in a name? Int J Gynecol Pathol. 2016;35(1):78–81.
20. Wu CH, Mao TL, Vang R, Ayhan A, Wang TL, Kurman RJ, Shih IM. Endocervical-type mucinous borderline tumors are related to endometrioid tumors based on mutation and loss of expression of ARID1A. Int J Gynecol Pathol. 2012;31(4):297–303.
21. Nakamura E, Sato Y, Moriguchi S, Yamashita A, Higo T, Asada Y. Ovarian seromucinous borderline tumor and clear cell carcinoma: an unusual combination. Case Rep Obstet Gynecol. 2015;2015:690891. Published online 2015 May 13. https://doi.org/10.1155/2015/690891.
22. Maeda D, Shih IM. Pathogenesis and the role of ARID1A mutation in endometriosis-related ovarian neoplasms. Adv Anat Pathol. 2013;20(1):45–52.
23. Kurata Y, Kido A, Moribata Y, Kameyama K, Himoto Y, Minamiguchi S, Konishi I, Togashi K. Diagnostic performance of MR imaging findings and quantitative values in the differentiation of seromucinous borderline tumour from endometriosis-related malignant ovarian tumour. Eur Radiol. 2017;27(4):1695–703. [Epub ahead of print].

Development of Breast Carcinoma in Relation to the Intrinsic Subtype

7

Takuya Moriya

Abstract

Breast cancer is a heterogeneous disease, both histologically and genetically. Various intrinsic subtypes with different biological characteristics have been proposed. The frequency and developmental pathways of each subtype vary. Thus, non-cancerous and borderline lesions that might be related to breast cancer were examined, and their links with distinct intrinsic subtypes of breast cancer were considered. In particular, the significance of the most potent precursors (non-obligate precursors) was evaluated.

Keywords

Breast · Carcinoma · Precursor lesion · Atypical hyperplasia · Pathology

7.1 Introduction

Breast carcinoma is the most common type of cancer among Japanese women. Approximately one eleventh of women suffer breast cancer during their lives. Females aged >40 years are recommended to undergo annual breast cancer screening examinations. Monthly self-checks are another important tool for detecting breast cancer earlier. Several risk factors for breast cancer have been reported, including early first menstruation, late menopause, nulliparity, obesity (especially after the menopause), a family history of breast cancer, a clinical history of benign breast disease, a history of endometrial cancer or ovarian tumor, therapeutic sex steroid hormone intake, and heavy alcohol drinking.

However, breast cancer is a heterogeneous disease, both morphologically and genetically. Most types of breast cancer are sex steroid hormone-dependent, but this is not the case for all types. So, some types of breast cancer might arise via different pathways from typical (the most frequent types, hormone-dependent) tumors, and they might also have different risk factors. In this chapter, the various intrinsic subtypes of breast carcinoma are examined, and the precursor and/or non-cancerous lesions related to each intrinsic subtype are discussed.

7.2 Intrinsic Subtypes of Breast Cancer

The various original intrinsic subtypes of breast cancer were based on molecular features. Perou et al. analyzed 496 genes in 65 breast cancer samples from 42 patients using a cDNA microarray and divided the samples into four clusters (luminal epithelial/estrogen receptor (ER), ErbB2 (also known as human epidermal growth factor receptor 2 [HER2]) overexpression, basal epithelial associated containing keratin 5 and 17, second basal epithelial-cell-enriched) [1]. Several subsequent studies employed different sets of genes to analyze varying numbers of patients, but five intrinsic subtypes became fixed (luminal A, luminal B, HER2+/ER-, basal-like, and normal breast-like) [2–4]. Among them, the significance of the normal breast-like subtype is disputed, as the contamination of normal breast tissue during clustering had not been adequately considered.

The other four intrinsic subtypes seemed to be based on ER, progesterone receptor (PgR), and HER2 expression, so immunohistochemical methods were widely used to assess the intrinsic subtype of breast cancer thereafter [4]. Tumors that are negative for ER, PgR, and HER2 are referred to as "triple negative." They tend to exhibit higher-grade histology and a worse prognosis than luminal-type tumors [5, 6]. Among triple-negative cancers, cytokeratin (CK)5/6 and/or epidermal growth factor receptor (EGFR)-positive cases are considered to belong to the basal-like phenotype [7], and the prognosis of such cases is much worse than that of non-basal-type triple-negative cancer. Subsequently, the claudin-

T. Moriya
Department of Pathology, Kawasaki Medical School, Kurashiki, Okayama, Japan
e-mail: tmoriya@med.kawasaki-m.ac.jp

T. Moriya (ed.), *Pathology of Female Cancers*, https://doi.org/10.1007/978-981-10-8606-9_7

low subtype, which displays stem cell and mesenchymal cell features, has been proposed [8]. In addition, a more precise system for subtyping breast cancer based on the optimal chemotherapy regimen has been proposed [9]. This classification includes two basal-like subtypes, an immunomodulatory subtype, a mesenchymal subtype, a mesenchymal stemlike subtype, and a luminal androgen receptor subtype. However, the claudin-low subtype and the latter six subtypes do not exhibit characteristic morphological features, and so they are not currently used in routine pathological practice. The 2015 St Gallen consensus meeting described a treatment-oriented pathological classification system for breast cancer based on ER, PgR, and HER2 expression; the Ki-67 labeling index; tumor size; lymph node status; histological grade; lymphovascular invasion; and multiparameter molecular markers [10].

Although most breast tumors belong to the luminal phenotype, the frequency of each intrinsic subtype might differ according to race. For example, the incidence of triple-negative breast cancer is much higher among African Americans than among Caucasian women in the United States [4], and it is much lower among Japanese [11]. If the pathways responsible for the development of breast cancer and precursor lesions vary between the different intrinsic subtypes, the incidence of benign breast diseases might also differ between races. However, no significant race-related differences in the incidence of benign breast disease or subsequent breast cancer were detected in several studies [12–14]. Additional studies, especially analyses of precise types of benign breast disease and related intrinsic subtypes, will be required.

7.3 Cellular Origin of Breast Carcinoma

Breast carcinoma basically arises from breast epithelial cells. Historically, it was considered that different tumors arise from the ductal and lobular epithelia (i.e., ductal carcinoma and lobular carcinoma); however, it is currently believed that both ductal carcinoma and lobular carcinoma are derived from the same epithelial tissue at terminal duct-lobular units. There has been speculation regarding epithelial development and its relationships with the various intrinsic subtypes of breast carcinoma [15] (Fig. 7.1). Normal mammary epithelial cells differentiate from stem cells into bipotent progenitor cells, and then further differentiate via two pathways, i.e., into myoepithelial and luminal cells. Most (probably almost all) breast carcinomas are derived from the stem cell/luminal cell lineage because myoepithelial carcinoma is extremely rare. Thus, theoretically the various intrinsic subtypes of

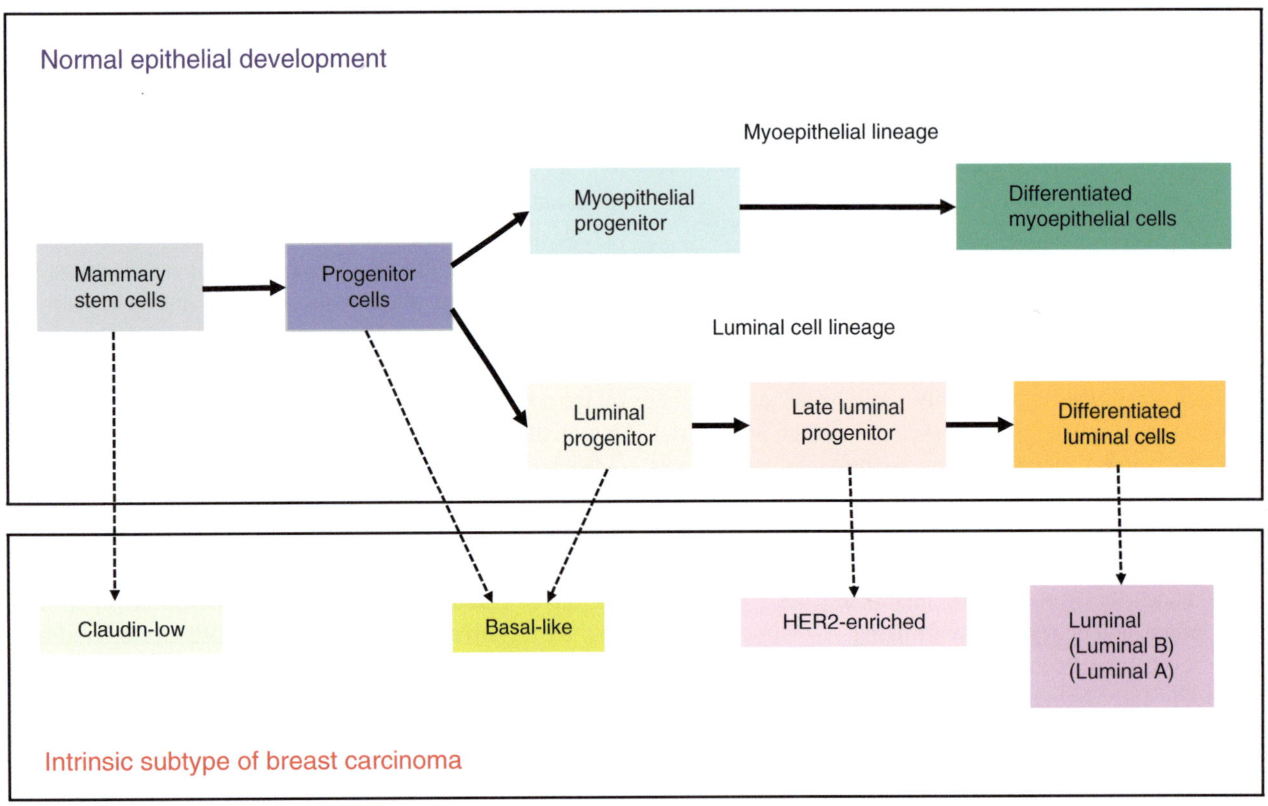

Fig. 7.1 Mammary epithelial development and its relationships with the various intrinsic subtypes of breast carcinoma. Each intrinsic subtype of breast cancer might be derived from cells from a different stage of normal mammary epithelial development

breast carcinomas might arise from cells exhibiting different degrees of luminal cell differentiation. Claudin-low-type cancer is derived from mammary stem cells; basal-like carcinoma is derived from more differentiated but bipotent/luminal progenitor cells; and luminal-type carcinomas are derived from the most differentiated luminal epithelial cells, which express steroid hormone receptors.

Applying this concept to the morphology of breast cancer, we should be aware of the immunohistochemical features of normal breast tissue (Fig. 7.2). The normal mammary duct contains both (luminal) epithelial and myoepithelial cells, which is called the biphasic (two-cell) pattern. The myoepithelial cells are located on the outer side of such ducts, and their nuclei are positive for p63. Luminal epithelial cells are positive for ER (and PgR), but do not exhibit diffuse positivity for ER [16, 17]. ER-negative cells are admixed in normal tissue, and the staining intensity of positive nuclei might vary. Myoepithelial cells and some luminal epithelial cells are positive for CK5/6 and CK14 and high-molecular-weight CK, and the latter cell type might be analogous to ER-negative epithelial cells.

The immunohistochemical expression patterns of breast epithelial lesions, including both benign and malignant lesions, might be strongly related to their cellular origins. For example, ductal hyperplasia is composed of a heterogeneous cell population and exhibits mosaic-like CK5/6, CK14, and ER expression patterns. On the other hand, atypical ductal hyperplasia (ADH) and low-grade ductal carcinoma in situ (DCIS) are uniformly negative for CK5/6 and CK14 and diffusely and strongly positive for the ER [18]. The latter lesions are considered to be neoplastic as well as monomorphous. In the same way, the immunohistochemical characteristics of breast carcinoma can be used as a basis for speculating on its cellular origin, and precursor lesions might display the same expression patterns as related tumors.

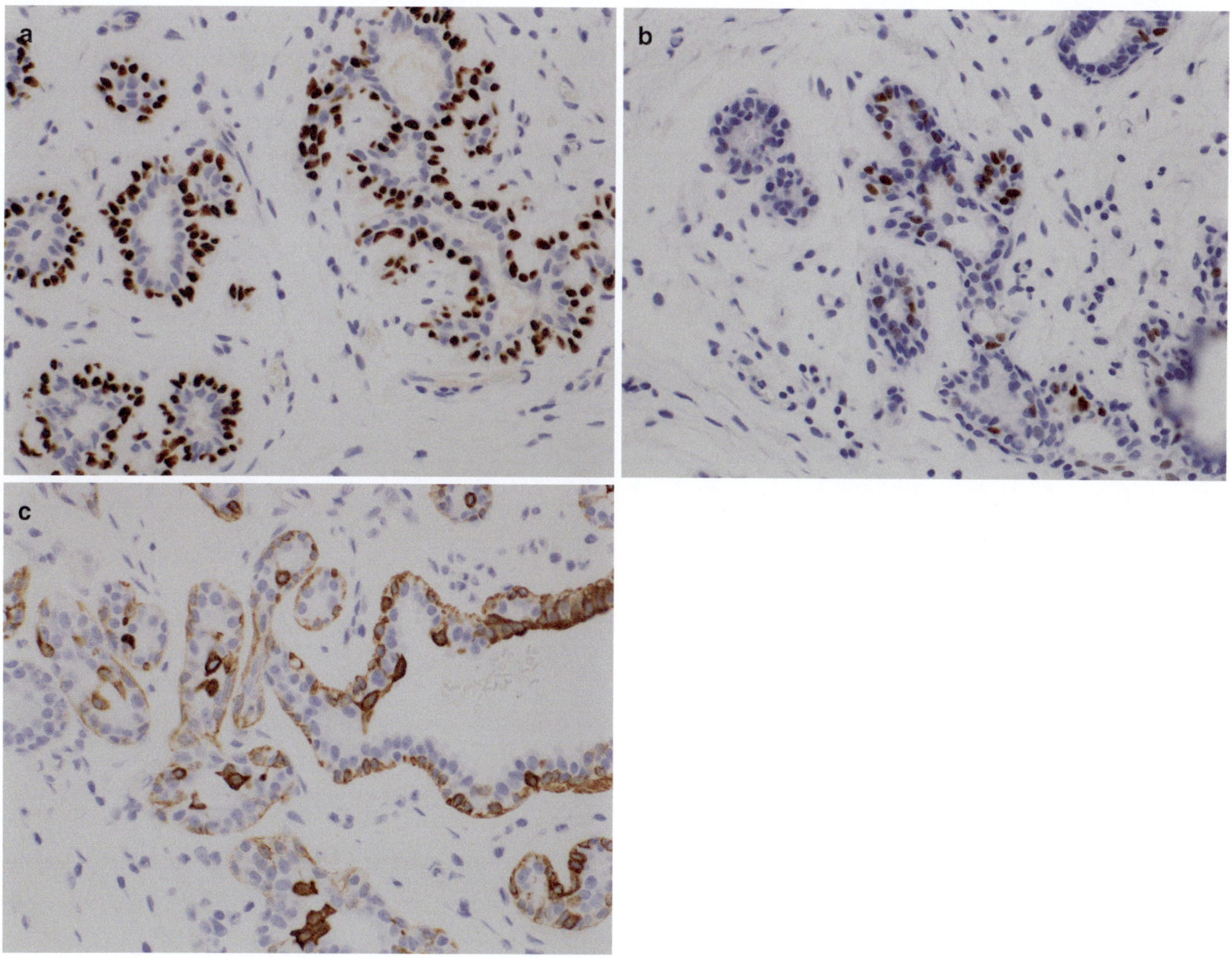

Fig. 7.2 Immunohistochemical features of normal mammary ducts. (**a**) The myoepithelial cells on the outer side of the mammary duct are positive for p63. (**b**) The luminal epithelium is positive for the ER, but its expression is not diffuse. (**c**) The luminal epithelial cells are heterogeneously positive for CK14, showing a mosaic-like staining pattern

7.4 Atypical Epithelial Lesions and Their Significance as Precursors

Atypical epithelial lesions include flat epithelial atypia (FEA), ADH, and lobular neoplasia (LN). LN includes atypical lobular hyperplasia (ALH) and lobular carcinoma in situ (LCIS), and clinically they are treated similarly. DCIS is the real precursor of invasive (ductal) carcinoma but is usually excluded from atypical lesions (even low-grade lesions).

In general, patients with atypical hyperplasia (ADH and LN) are considered to be at risk of developing invasive breast carcinoma. Females with these lesions are at higher risk of developing breast cancer in both the ipsilateral and contralateral breasts in the future. There have been many cohort studies examining these lesions [13, 19–23]. Some studies have shown that the extent and type of atypical hyperplasia influence the risk of cancer [21], but this is still controversial, probably due to differences in study designs [24].

In one study, it was reported that ADH and LN were associated with ipsilateral, stage I, ER-positive invasive cancer [21]; thus, they might be related to low-grade luminal-type breast cancer. It is possible to consider ADH as a non-obligate breast cancer precursor, but by definition ADH is a small lesion (within two ducts or with a diameter of ≤2 mm) [25], and so it is often incidentally found in biopsy specimens (Fig. 7.3). At least some ADH lesions can be completely removed via a biopsy examination. However, the natural history of ADH lesions is still unclear. In addition, a study conducted in Egypt detected the overexpression of HER2/neu in ADH and DCIS and found that these lesions were related to HER2-positive invasive cancer [26]. In the latter study, it was reported that four of six sclerosing adenosis/ADH lesions exhibited scores of 3+ during immunohistochemical staining of HER2. However, 26% of non-atypical epithelial lesions (fibrocystic disease/usual ductal hyperplasia) were also HER2-positive, which is an unexpectedly high incidence. Further studies are required to resolve various technical/racial problems related to these findings.

LN (Fig. 7.4), even LCIS, is absolutely a high-risk lesion in terms of its association with breast cancer, and the risk is same for both invasive ductal carcinoma and invasive lobular carcinoma and for both breasts [27, 28]. However, except for pleomorphic LN, there is no evidence that LN (ADH and LCIS) is a direct precursor of invasive carcinoma (especially the lobular type).

FEA, another type of lesion involving epithelial atypia (Fig. 7.5), might be associated with ADH, LN, and/or carcinoma in the same breast. It is not a strong independent risk factor for breast cancer, but it might be significantly associated with ADH/ALH [29]. So, some researchers consider that FEA could be a non-obligate precursor of ADH [25]. However, FEA is a risk factor for both breasts, but does not raise the local risk of developing breast cancer [30].

In summary, ADH, LN, and FEA are considered to be risk factors for the development of breast carcinoma, but there is no clear evidence from long-term follow-up studies to indicate that they directly transition into (invasive) carcinoma.

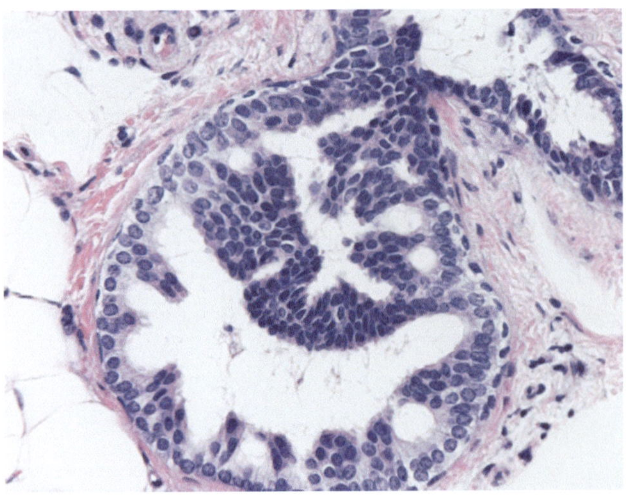

Fig. 7.3 Atypical ductal hyperplasia. These lesions exhibit a similar morphology to low-grade DCIS, but do not fully satisfy the associated criteria. They are usually small

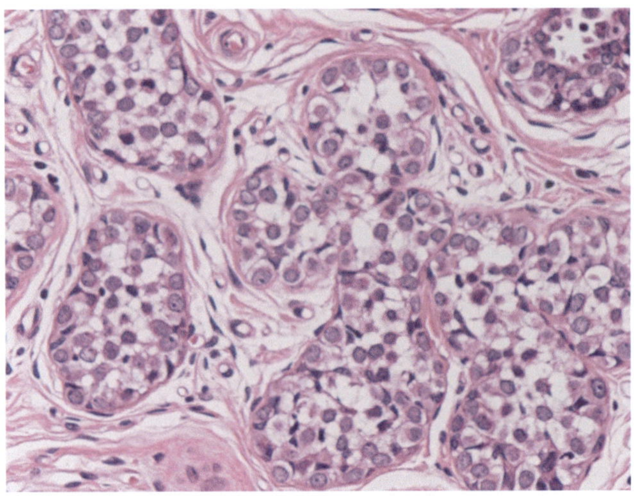

Fig. 7.4 Lobular neoplasia. Uniform and dyscohesive epithelial cells are found located within duct-lobular units

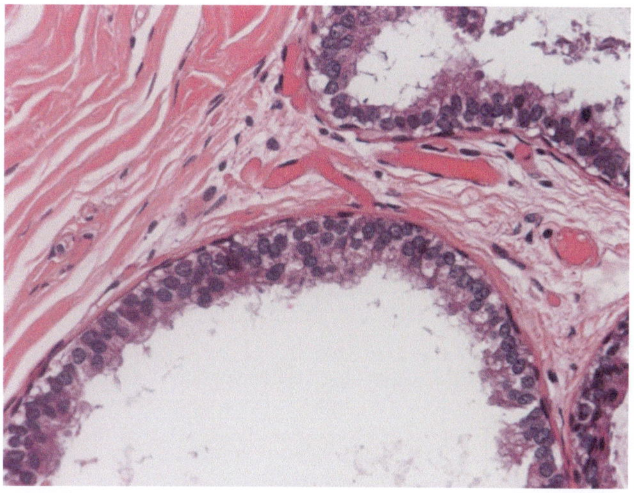

Fig. 7.5 Flat epithelial atypia. Uniform, round nuclei are stratified on small dilated ducts

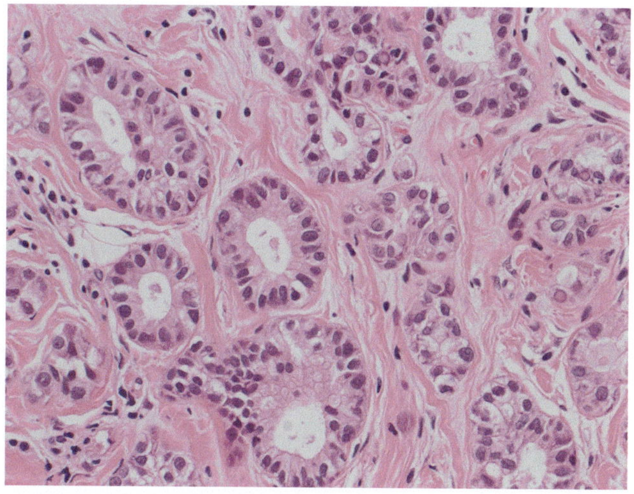

Fig. 7.6 Atypical microglandular hyperplasia. These lesions lack myoepithelial cells, and their epithelial cells are positive for S-100. Atypical nuclei with some mitotic figures are seen

7.5 Breast Lesions that Coexist with Breast Carcinoma as Possible Precursors

There are several non-cancerous lesions that frequently coexist with breast cancer. They are often found at the time of excision and might act as potent non-obligate precursors of tumors.

It is well known that associations exist among columnar cell lesions (including FEA), LN, and tubular carcinoma (well-differentiated, luminal A-type invasive carcinoma), which are sometimes called the "Rosen triad" [31]. Although the genetic abnormalities shared by these three lesions have been clarified, the roles of LN and FEA as precursors have already been discussed. Mucocele-like lesions (MLL) might also accompany luminal A-type breast cancer. They are frequently associated with ADH and are sometimes related to low-grade DCIS or invasive carcinoma (especially mucinous carcinoma). However, MLL without epithelial atypia does not increase the relative risk of breast cancer. Thus, cancer development is related to atypical lesions, rather than to MLL itself [32, 33].

Microglandular adenosis (MGA) is a rare lesion, which is often associated with high histological grade and triple-negative invasive breast carcinoma. There are several articles describing invasive carcinoma arising in MGA. For example, atypical MGA has been reported to coexist (Fig. 7.6) with in situ and invasive carcinoma and often expresses the S-100 protein [32, 33]. The cancers associated with MGA include metaplastic (matrix-producing) carcinoma and acinar cell carcinoma, although these histological types might be quite rare, and MGA probably does not explain the occurrence of the majority of triple-negative carcinomas.

Conclusion

The progression pathways of breast cancer are heterogeneous and involve various lineages. Different grades of carcinoma (i.e., low- and high-grade) and/or different intrinsic subtypes might have different precursors. Several non-obligate precursors of breast cancer have been proposed, and some of them are high-risk lesions for breast cancer. They are associated with low-grade/luminal A-like carcinomas and are referred to as the "low-grade breast neoplasia family" according to clinicopathological and genetic studies [34]. However, many of the links between non-cancerous precursors and carcinoma (both in situ and invasive) remain unclear (Fig. 7.7). We still do not know how many carcinomas occur de novo or how often low-grade carcinomas progress to become high-grade carcinomas. For the sake of prevention, further studies will be necessary to clarify the precursor lesions that directly progress into cancer in the future, rather than simply detecting high-risk lesions as indirect (but useful) markers. Genetic studies, which were not covered in detail in this chapter, are also indispensable.

Acknowledgment This work was supported by JSPS KAKENHI Grant Grant-in-Aid for Scientific Research (C), Numbers JP25460467 and JP16K08701.

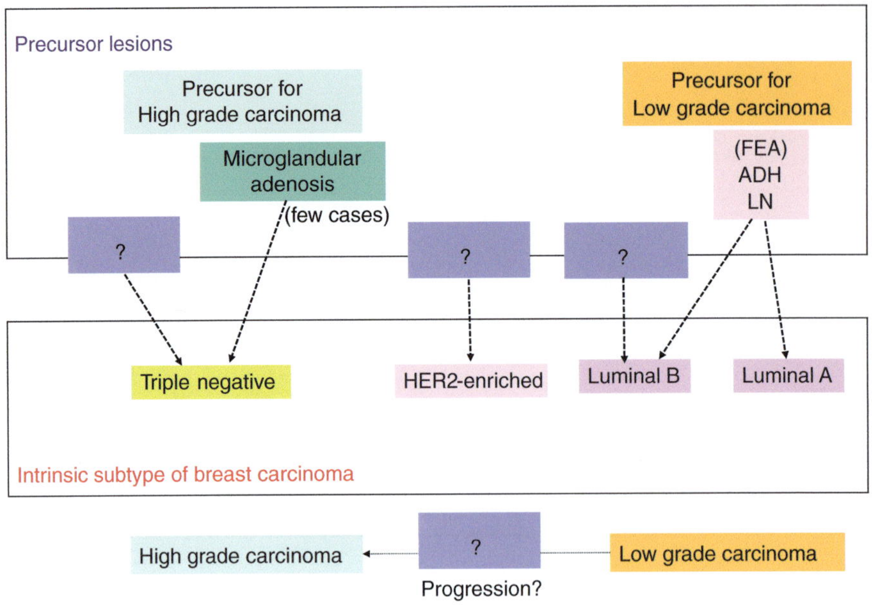

Fig. 7.7 Possible non-obligate precursors and their relationships with the various intrinsic subtypes of breast carcinoma. The relationships between precursor lesions and the corresponding intrinsic subtypes of breast cancer are shown, but many of these relationships remain unclear. In addition, the significance of the progression of low-grade cancer to high-grade cancer has not been fully elucidated

References

1. Perou CM, Sørlie T, Eisen MB, van de Rijn M, Jeffrey SS, Rees CA, Pollack JR, Ross DT, Johnsen H, Akslen LA, Fluge O, Pergamenschikov A, Williams C, Zhu SX, Lønning PE, Børresen-Dale AL, Brown PO, Botstein D. Molecular portraits of human breast tumours. Nature. 2000;406(6797):747–52.
2. Sørlie T, Perou CM, Tibshirani R, Aas T, Geisler S, Johnsen H, Hastie T, Eisen MB, van de Rijn M, Jeffrey SS, Thorsen T, Quist H, Matese JC, Brown PO, Botstein D, Lønning PE, Børresen-Dale AL. Gene expression patterns of breast carcinomas distinguish tumor subclasses with clinical implications. Proc Natl Acad Sci U S A. 2001;98(19):10869–74.
3. Sorlie T, Tibshirani R, Parker J, Hastie T, Marron JS, Nobel A, Deng S, Johnsen H, Pesich R, Geisler S, Demeter J, Perou CM, Lønning PE, Brown PO, Børresen-Dale AL, Botstein D. Repeated observation of breast tumor subtypes in independent gene expression data sets. Proc Natl Acad Sci U S A. 2003;100(14):8418–23. Epub 2003 Jun 26.
4. Carey LA, Perou CM, Livasy CA, Dressler LG, Cowan D, Conway K, Karaca G, Troester MA, Tse CK, Edmiston S, Deming SL, Geradts J, Cheang MC, Nielsen TO, Moorman PG, Earp HS, Millikan RC. Race, breast cancer subtypes, and survival in the Carolina Breast Cancer Study. JAMA. 2006;295(21):2492–502.
5. Reis-Filho JS, Tutt AN. Triple negative tumours: a critical review. Histopathology. 2008;52(1):108–18.
6. Rakha EA, El-Sayed ME, Green AR, Lee AH, Robertson JF, Ellis IO. Prognostic markers in triple-negative breast cancer. Cancer. 2007;109(1):25–32.
7. Tischkowitz M, Brunet JS, Bégin LR, Huntsman DG, Cheang MC, Akslen LA, Nielsen TO, Foulkes WD. Use of immunohistochemical markers can refine prognosis in triple negative breast cancer. BMC Cancer. 2007;7:134.
8. Prat A, Perou CM. Deconstructing the molecular portraits of breast cancer. Mol Oncol. 2011;5(1):5–23.
9. Mayer IA, Abramson VG, Lehmann BD, Pietenpol JA. New strategies for triple-negative breast cancer—deciphering the heterogeneity. Clin Cancer Res. 2014;20(4):782–90.
10. Coates AS, Winer EP, Goldhirsch A, Gelber RD, Gnant M, Piccart-Gebhart M, Thürlimann B, Senn HJ, Members P. Tailoring therapies—improving the management of early breast cancer: St Gallen International Expert Consensus on the Primary Therapy of Early Breast Cancer 2015. Ann Oncol. 2015;26(8):1533–46.
11. Kurebayashi J, Moriya T, Ishida T, Hirakawa H, Kurosumi M, Akiyama F, Kinoshita T, Takei H, Takahashi K, Ikeda M, Nakashima K. The prevalence of intrinsic subtypes and prognosis in breast cancer patients of different races. Breast. 2007;16(Suppl 2):S72–7.
12. Worsham MJ, Abrams J, Raju U, Kapke A, Lu M, Cheng J, Mott D, Wolman SR. Breast cancer incidence in a cohort of women with benign breast disease from a multiethnic, primary health care population. Breast J. 2007;13(2):115–21.
13. Cote ML, Ruterbusch JJ, Alosh B, Bandyopadhyay S, Kim E, Albashiti B, Sharaf Aldeen B, Radisky DC, Frost MH, Visscher DW, Hartmann LC, Nassar WH, Ali-Femhi R. Benign breast disease and the risk of subsequent breast cancer in African American women. Cancer Prev Res (Phila). 2012;5(12):1375–80.
14. Newman LA, Stark A, Chitale D, Pepe M, Longton G, Worsham MJ, Nathanson SD, Miller P, Bensenhaver JM, Proctor E, Swain M, Patriotis C, Engstrom PF. Association between benign breast disease in African American and white American women and subsequent triple-negative breast cancer. JAMA Oncol. 2017;3(8):1102–6.
15. Perou CM. Molecular stratification of triple-negative breast cancers. Oncologist. 2010;15(Suppl 5):39–48.
16. Oh H, Eliassen AH, Wang M, Smith-Warner SA, Beck AH, Schnitt SJ, Collins LC, Connolly JL, Montaser-Kouhsari L, Polyak K, Tamimi RM. Expression of estrogen receptor, progesterone receptor, and Ki67 in normal breast tissue in relation to subsequent risk of breast cancer. NPJ Breast Cancer. 2016;2:pii: 16032. https://doi.org/10.1038/npjbcancer.2016.32. Epub 2016 Oct 26.
17. Woolcott CG, SenGupta SK, Hanna WM, Aronson KJ. Estrogen and progesterone receptor levels in nonneoplastic breast epithelium of breast cancer cases versus benign breast biopsy controls. BMC Cancer. 2008;8:130. https://doi.org/10.1186/1471-2407-8-130.
18. Moriya T, Kanomata N, Kozuka Y, Hirakawa H, Kimijima I, Kimura M, Watanabe M, Sasano H, Ishida T, Ohuchi N, Kurebayashi J, Sonoo H. Molecular morphological approach to the pathological

study of development and advancement of human breast cancer. Med Mol Morphol. 2010;43(2):67–73.
19. Dupont WD, Page DL. Risk factors for breast cancer in women with proliferative breast disease. N Engl J Med. 1985;312(3):146–51.
20. Dyrstad SW, Yan Y, Fowler AM, Colditz GA. Breast cancer risk associated with benign breast disease: systematic review and meta-analysis. Breast Cancer Res Treat. 2015;149(3):569–75.
21. Donaldson AR, McCarthy C, Goraya S, Pederson HJ, Sturgis CD, Grobmyer SR, Calhoun BC. Breast cancer risk associated with atypical hyperplasia and lobular carcinoma in situ initially diagnosed on core-needle biopsy. Cancer. 2017;124:459. https://doi.org/10.1002/cncr.31061. [Epub ahead of print].
22. McEvoy MP, Coopey SB, Mazzola E, Buckley J, Belli A, Polubriaginof F, Merrill AL, Tang R, Garber JE, Smith BL, Gadd MA, Specht MC, Guidi AJ, Roche CA, Hughes KS. Breast cancer risk and follow-up recommendations for young women diagnosed with atypical hyperplasia and lobular carcinoma in situ (LCIS). Ann Surg Oncol. 2015;22(10):3346–9.
23. Dion L, Racin A, Brousse S, Beltjens F, Cauchois A, Levêque J, Coutant C, Lavoué V. Atypical epithelial hyperplasia of the breast: state of the art. Expert Rev Anticancer Ther. 2016;16(9):943–53.
24. Collins LC, Aroner SA, Connolly JL, Colditz GA, Schnitt SJ, Tamimi RM. Breast cancer risk by extent and type of atypical hyperplasia: an update from the Nurses' Health Studies. Cancer. 2016;122(4):515–20.
25. Bombonati A, Sgroi DC. The molecular pathology of breast cancer progression. J Pathol. 2011;223(2):307–17.
26. Daoud SA, Ismail WM, Abdelhamid MS, Nabil TM, Daoud SA. Possible prognostic role of HER2/Neu in ductal carcinoma in situ and atypical ductal proliferative lesions of the breast. Asian Pac J Cancer Prev. 2016;17(8):3733–6.
27. Fisher ER, Land SR, Fisher B, Mamounas E, Gilarski L, Wolmark N. Pathologic findings from the National Surgical Adjuvant Breast and Bowel Project: twelve-year observations concerning lobular carcinoma in situ. Cancer. 2004;100(2):238–44.
28. Chuba PJ, Hamre MR, Yap J, Severson RK, Lucas D, Shamsa F, Aref A. Bilateral risk for subsequent breast cancer after lobular carcinoma-in-situ: analysis of surveillance, epidemiology, and end results data. J Clin Oncol. 2005;23(24):5534–41.
29. Boulos FI, Dupont WD, Schuyler PA, Sanders ME, Page DL, Fedda FA, Simpson JF. Clinicopathologic characteristics of carcinomas that develop after a biopsy containing columnar cell lesions: evidence against a precursor role. Cancer. 2012;118(9):2372–7.
30. Said SM, Visscher DW, Nassar A, Frank RD, Vierkant RA, Frost MH, Ghosh K, Radisky DC, Hartmann LC, Degnim AC. Flat epithelial atypia and risk of breast cancer: a Mayo cohort study. Cancer. 2015;121(10):1548–55.
31. Brandt SM, Young GQ, Hoda SA. The "Rosen Triad": tubular carcinoma, lobular carcinoma in situ, and columnar cell lesions. Adv Anat Pathol. 2008;15(3):140–6.
32. Meares AL, Frank RD, Degnim AC, Vierkant RA, Frost MH, Hartmann LC, Winham SJ, Visscher DW. Mucocele-like lesions of the breast: a clinical outcome and histologic analysis of 102 cases. Hum Pathol. 2016;49:33–8.
33. Zhang G, Ataya D, L Lebda P, Calhoun BC. Mucocele-like lesions diagnosed on breast core biopsy: low risk of upgrade and subsequent carcinoma. Breast J. 2017. https://doi.org/10.1111/tbj.12929. [Epub ahead of print].
34. Lopez-Garcia MA, Geyer FC, Lacroix-Triki M, Marchió C, Reis-Filho JS. Breast cancer precursors revisited: molecular features and progression pathways. Histopathology. 2010;57(2):171–92.

Morphological and Molecular Approaches to Breast Cancer Risk Assessment

8

Shinobu Masuda

Abstract

Data on risk factors for breast cancer has been emerging from epidemiological, morphological, and molecular analysis. Here, two inherent high-risk factors, germline mutations and family history, are reviewed in addition to moderate-risk factors related to pathological findings, including atypical ductal hyperplasia and atypical lobular hyperplasia. Concrete clinical evidence abounds for the relationship between exposure to estrogen and breast cancer; however, the mechanisms how estrogens and estrogen receptors (ERα, ERβ) are involved in carcinogenesis of breast cancer have not been fully clarified. These estrogen receptors are discussed as risk factors in this chapter. Finally, recent molecular investigations reveal that genetic alterations occur even in the mammary gland that lacks morphological atypical features. The significance of such genetic alterations without histological atypia has not yet been clarified. The biological and clinical significance of this phenomenon is expected to be elucidated for better prevention and treatment in the near future.

Keywords

Risk factor · Breast cancer · Atypical hyperplasia · Estrogen receptor

8.1 Introduction

Identifying risk factors for breast cancer is closely related to investigating carcinogenesis, as well as to preventing and treating carcinoma for better prognosis. Historically, risk factors have been demonstrated epidemiologically; recent evidence has emerged from morphological and molecular analysis. Risk factors for breast cancer are inherent and the individual cannot change them, and they are often related to lifestyle; other risk factors encompass both susceptibility and lifestyle (Table 8.1). The first group of factors includes female sex, an inherited germline mutation, and a positive family history. The second group of factors is alcohol intake, body mass index, and hormone replacement therapy with estrogen and progesterone. The last group of factors is prolonged exposure to estrogen (early menarche, late menopause), age at first childbirth, past history of breast cancer and various histological changes, and radiation exposure.

In this chapter, high-risk factors related to germline mutations and family history will be described followed by moderate-risk histologic and morphological factors. Then, the risks associated with estrogen exposure and estrogen receptors will be reviewed, and numerical and structural chromosomal alterations and epigenetic changes even in the morphologically normal mammary gland will be discussed.

8.2 Risk Assessment by Germline Mutations and Family History

Genetic linkage studies have demonstrated that the *BRCA1* gene, located on 17q21, is related to the early onset of breast cancer and/or ovarian cancer [1, 2], and it was shown to be responsible for almost all familial breast cancer [3]. The cDNA sequence and structure of *BRCA1* were found to consist of 22 exons encoding a 1863-residue protein [4]. *BRCA1* has critical roles in DNA repair, especially with the activation of double-strand break repair and/or homologous recombination.

An early study in families with multiple cases of breast cancer reported extremely high relative risk of lifetime breast cancer for *BRCA1* mutation carriers. In this series, relative risk for women with *BRCA1* germline mutation, compared with risk in the general population (England and Wales 1978–1982), was >200-fold for women aged under 40 years and 15-fold for women aged 60–69 years. Estimated cumu-

S. Masuda
Department of Pathology, Nihon University School of Medicine, Tokyo, Japan
e-mail: masuda.shinobu@nihon-u.ac.jp

T. Moriya (ed.), *Pathology of Female Cancers*, https://doi.org/10.1007/978-981-10-8606-9_8

Table 8.1 Risk factors for breast cancer

Risk factor	Category at risk	Comparison category	Relative risk	Reference
Inherent factors				
Germline mutation	See Table 8.2			
Family history	First-degree relative ≥50 years with postmenopausal BC	No	1.8	[98]
	First-degree relative with premenopausal BC	No	3.3	
	Second-degree relative with BC	No	1.5	
	Two first-degree relatives with BC	No	3.6	
Lifestyle-related factors				
Alcohol intake	Two drinks per day	Nondrinker	1.2	[99]
Body mass index	80th percentile, age ≥55	20th percentile	1.2	[100]
Hormone RT	Current user for ≥5 years	Never used	1.3	[101]
Others				
Age (years)	≥65	<65	5.8	[102]
Prolonged exposure to estrogen				
Early menarche	<12 years	>15 years	1.3	[39]
Late menopause	>55 years	<45 years	1.2–1.5	[36, 39]
Age at first childbirth	Nulliparous or first child after 30	First child before 20	1.7–1.9	[37, 38, 103]
Past history				
Invasive breast cancer	Present	Absent	6.8	[104, 105]
LCIS	Present	Absent	16.4	[106, 107]
DCIS	Present	Absent	17.3	
Hyperplasia with atypia and positive family history		No hyperplasia and negative family history	11	[108]
Hyperplasia with atypia	Present	Absent	5.3	[108]
Hyperplasia without atypia	Present	Absent	1.9	[108]
Radiation exposure				
Repeated fluoroscopy		No exposure	1.6	[109, 110]
Radiation therapy for Hodgkin's disease		No exposure	5.2	

BC breast cancer; *RT* replacement therapy; *LCIS* lobular carcinoma in situ; *DCIS* ductal carcinoma in situ

lative risk of breast cancer was 54.2% at age 60 and 85.0% at age 70 [5]. These high-risk results were estimated from data on families with multiple cases of breast cancer that may be enriched for the *BRCA1* mutation. Some studies evaluated accumulated data that included a more general population [6] and performed a meta-analysis [7]. Similar to the previous study, cumulative risk at age 70 for *BRCA1* mutation carriers was reported as 65% [6] and 57% [7] for breast cancer and 39% [6] and 40% [7] for ovarian cancer. For *BRCA2* mutation carriers, cumulative risk at age 70 was also similarly reported as 45% [6] and 40% [7] for breast cancer and 11% [6] and 18% [7] for ovarian cancer (Table 8.2).

Estimating breast cancer risk can be conducted with several risk assessment models [8–15]. The Gail model [8], based on the Breast Cancer Risk Assessment Tool, was designed for women without specific high-risk factors. Minimal information about family history for first-degree relatives is required to use this model. The Claus model [15], International Breast Cancer Intervention Study (IBIS) model [11], BRCAPRO model [10], and BOADICEA model [12–14] are for women at high risk; these models all require multigenerational family history of breast and ovarian cancer. Each model was designed based on different risk factors, so the risk is estimated differently for each individual.

8.3 Risk Assessment Related to Pathological Findings

8.3.1 Atypical Hyperplasia

Breast cancer shows a variety of histopathological features ranging from benign to malignant. It is often difficult to definitively categorize a lesion as benign or malignant, and such a lesion would be categorized as intermediate. The designation and definition of these lesions are debatable; "atypical hyperplasia" is the most commonly used term and comprises atypical ductal hyperplasia (ADH) and atypical lobular hyperplasia (ALH). The general consensus is that ADH is "a proliferative lesion that fulfills some but not all criteria for a diagnosis of DCIS" (ductal carcinoma in situ) [16]. Certain definitions include quantitative estimation,

Table 8.2 *BRCA1* and *BRCA2* gene alterations as risk factors

BRCA1	Cumulative risk						Relative risk[a]		
Age (years)	Breast cancer (%)			Ovarian cancer (%)			Breast cancer (%)		Ovarian cancer (%)
Reference	[5]	[6]	[7]	[5]	[6]	[7]	[5]	[6]	[6]
20–29								17	1
30–39	3.2			0.2			>200	33	49
40–49	19.1			0.6				32	68
50–59	50.8			22.7				18	31
60–69	54.2			29.8			15	14	50
70	85.0	65	57	63.3	39	40			

BRCA2	Cumulative risk				Relative risk[a]	
Age	Breast cancer (%)		Ovarian cancer (%)		Breast cancer (%)	Ovarian cancer (%)
Reference	[6]	[7]	[6]	[7]	[6]	[6]
20–29					19	1.0
30–39					16	1.0
40–49					9.9	6.3
50–59					12	19
60–69					11	8.4
70	45	40	11	18		

[a]Compared with incidence for England and Wales in 1973–1977

which part of description was emphasized and widely spread. For example, ADH is defined either as a proliferative lesion involving fewer than two duct spaces even if the abnormality is qualitatively consistent with DCIS [17] or as foci measuring <2 mm regardless of the number of affected duct cross sections, even if the individual ducts qualify as DCIS [18]. Rosen raised concerns about the strict application of such arbitrary definitions in practical clinical settings; however, lesion size could be considered in making a diagnosis, and these definitions are useful in research settings such as a single institution or a homogenous group [16]. Diagnosis of ADH has also been made from qualitative features including nuclear grade, mitotic activity, architectural structure, presence of necrosis, and associated proliferative lesions. If the lesion has a DCIS growth pattern in association with usual hyperplastic changes, it may be diagnosed as ADH. In spite of these considerations over definitions, the criteria by Page et al. [17] has been applied for the risk assessment studies discussed in the following paragraph.

The risk of ADH for breast cancer was reported as 4.4-fold by Page et al. in the Nashville Breast Cohort [17]. Subsequently, several groups reported increased risk of atypical hyperplasia (ductal and lobular) for breast cancer, including a retrospective cohort study by Mayo Clinic with an incidence ratio of 4.34 [19], the case-control Nurses' Health Study with an incidence ratio of 3.7 [20], the Henry Ford group [21], and a task force of the Japan Breast Cancer Society [22].

When considering the histological type of atypical hyperplasia (i.e., ADH and ALH), no obvious significant differences in incidence ratio have been reported (Table 8.3).

Table 8.3 Atypical hyperplasia as a risk factor

Histological type	No. of patients	Relative risk (95% CI)	*p* value	Later breast cancer
Mayo Clinic		SIR [19, 111][a]	0.54	
ADH	300	3.93 (3.00–5.06)		78% ductal, 22% lobular
ALH	327	4.76 (3.74–5.97)		77% ductal, 23% lobular
Atypical D and L	32	4.36 (1.75–8.96)		
Henry Ford		IRR [112][b]		
ADH	179	5.0 (2.3–11.0)		
ALH	67	3.2 (0.83–12.4)		
SEER cohort		SIR [23][c]		
LCIS	4853	7.1 (6.6–7.6)		49.7% ductal, 23.1% lobular

ADH atypical ductal hyperplasia; *ALH* atypical lobular hyperplasia; *atypical D and L* atypical ductal and lobular hyperplasia; *LCIS* lobular carcinoma in situ

[a]A retrospective cohort study comparing observed number of breast cancer events to those expected based on the Iowa SEER data (standardized incident ratio, SIR)

[b]A retrospective cohort study with incidence rate ratio (IRR). IRR is the ratio of incidence rates (IR) in those exposed to that of those unexposed, and IR is number of new cases divided by person years at risk

[c]A population-based study with standardized incident ratio (SIR) comparing observed rates with expected rates

In the Mayo Clinic cohort [19], the incidence ratio of ALH although relatively higher (4.76) than that of ADH (3.93) was not significantly higher and was not consistent with the findings in the Henry Ford group [21]. For lobular carcinoma in situ, the minimum risk of developing invasive breast carcinoma was calculated to be 7.1% at 10 years by analysis using Surveillance, Epidemiology, and End Results (SEER) data [23]. Interestingly, the histologic type of late-occurring breast cancer was predominantly ductal, even in patients with ALH as the initial lesion.

Whether or not extent of ADH and ALH is an increased risk factor for breast cancer is debatable. In 2007, Degnim et al. reported that the extent of atypical hyperplasia was related to increased risk in the Mayo Cohort [24]. This was confirmed again in the Mayo (n = 708) and Nashville (n = 466) cohorts in 2016. Relative risks of ADH with 1, 2, and ≥ 3 foci were 2.61, 5.21, and 6.36, respectively (p = 0.006 for linear trend), and ALH with 1, 2, and ≥ 3 foci were 2.56, 3.50, and 6.79 (p = 0.001 for linear trend) [25]. However, another group reported that the respective odds ratio of atypical hyperplasia with 1, 2, and ≥ 3 foci was 3.8, 4.5, and 5.3 with an increasing tendency, but there was no statistical significance (p = 0.22) [26]. Possible reasons for these discrepancies were selection bias due to methodological and sample size differences [27] and differences in criteria for diagnosing atypical hyperplasia [28]. Collaborative studies will help explain the reasons for these discrepancies, circulate information about these pathological criteria, and clarify the clinical significance of extent of atypical hyperplasia as a risk factor for breast cancer.

Further studies on family history in patients with atypical hyperplasia by Page et al. [17] reported that incidence ratio differed between groups with and without family histology in the Nashville Breast Cohort, but no other cohort studies have supported these findings (Table 8.4). The presence of atypical hyperplasia is considered to already reflect the risk inherent in family history.

Table 8.4 Family history as a risk factor

Family history	No. of patients	Relative risk (95% CI)	p value
Nashville Breast Cohort		RR [17][a]	
Yes	39	8.9 (4.8–17)	
No	193	3.5 (2.3–5.5)	
Mayo Clinic		SIR [19, 113][b]	0.23
None	372	3.91 (3.05–4.94)	
Weak	151	5.54 (3.93–7.57)	
Strong	106	4.19 (2.68–6.23)	
Nurses' Health Study		Adjusted OR [114][c]	0.57
Present	62	5.37 (3.01–9.58)	
Absent	194	4.38 (2.93–6.55)	

[a]A retrospective cohort study with relative risk (RR) in women from Atlanta, Georgia, in the Third National Cancer Society Survey controlled for age and number of years at risk

[b]A retrospective cohort study with standardized incident ratio (SIR) comparing observed number of breast cancer events to those expected based on the Iowa SEER data

[c]A case-control study with odds ratio (OR) adjusted for age at breast cancer diagnosis, year of benign breast biopsy, number of years of follow-up, age at menarche, age at first birth, body mass index, menopausal status, type of menopause and recency, and duration of postmenopausal hormone use between case and control

8.3.2 Histological Findings With or Without Atypical Hyperplasia (Table 8.5)

Flat epithelial atypia (FEA) is another type of epithelial proliferative lesion that cannot be simply categorized as benign or malignant. FEA is the most atypical lesion in a group of columnar cell alteration of lobules. Said et al. examined 11,591 women in the Mayo Benign Breast Disease (BBD) Cohort followed by excisional biopsy that consisted of 11,309 samples without FEA and 282 samples with FEA (2.4%). They found that the standardized incident ratio (SIR) of PDWA was 1.90 for samples without FEA and 2.04 for samples with FEA (p = 0.76) and that of atypical hyperplasia was 4.23 and 4.74, respectively (p = 0.59). Thus, FEA did not pose additional risk for proliferative disease without atypical hyperplasia (PDWA) or atypical hyperplasia [29].

Sclerosing adenosis (SA) is a common benign lesion with histologically complex features of increased fibrosis and enlarged distorted lobules. SA was detected in 27.8% of the

Table 8.5 Histologic findings as risk factors

	Total	Absent	Present	p value
Flat epithelial atypia [29]				
Number of patients	11,591	11,309	282	
SIR	Univariate	1.00	2.29	<0.001
	Multivariate	1.00	1.12	0.4781
With PDWA (n = 3736)		1.90	2.04	0.76
With AH (n = 597)		4.23	4.74	0.59
Sclerosing adenosis [30]				
Number of patients	13,434	9701	3733	
SIR		1.52	2.10	<0.0001
With NP (n = 8449)		1.34	1.39	0.7840
With PDWA (n = 4285)		1.99	1.97	0.9514
With AH (n = 700)		4.16	4.76	0.4206
Radial sclerosing complex [32]				
Number of patients	9262	8823	439	
SIR				
With PDWA (n = 2693)		1.57	1.88	0.29
With AH (n = 325)		3.97	2.81	0.33
Mucocele-like lesion [35]				
Number of patients	13,412	13,310	102	
SIR		1.63	2.28	0.255
With NP (n = 8449)		1.29	2.63	0.269
With PDWA (n = 4267)		1.94	3.18	0.943
With AH (n = 696)		4.30	1.37	0.413

NP no proliferative change; *PDWA* proliferative disease with atypia; *AH* atypical hyperplasia; *SIR* standardized incident ratio comparing observed number of breast cancer events to those expected based on the Iowa SEER data

BBD cohort (n = 13,434, 1967–2001) and was far more frequent than FEA. SIR was 1.52 and 2.10 in the SA-absent and SA-present groups, respectively ($p < 0.0001$) [30]. However, it was unclear whether the presence or absence of SA posed no increased risk for stratified groups with no proliferative changes (NP), PDWA, or atypical hyperplasia.

Radial scarring, originally reported by Hamperl et al., is a lesion that "consists of a hyalinized sclerotic center containing abundant elastic and elastoid masses. These radiate into the periphery and enclose lobuli which reveal epithelial proliferation varying from simple hyperplasia with epithelial villi to the rather rare true papillomas" [31]. The lesion is, however, not a true "scar" following some traumatic lesion, and thus radial sclerosing complex is proposed as a more suitable term. The presence of radial scars was not correlated to increase of SIR in the BBD cohort (n = 9262, 1967–1991) for breast cancer [32].

Mucocele-like lesions were originally reported as benign lesions that showed mucin extravasation into the stroma surrounding dilated ducts [33]. Epithelial cells lining dilated ducts vary from single layered without atypia, hyperplastic proliferative lesion with atypia, to carcinoma in situ [34]. The presence of mucocele-like lesions has not yet been shown to be a significant risk factor for breast cancer [35].

8.4 Risk Assessment Related to Reproductive Factors

Exposure to estrogen is related to breast cancer occurrence [36]. The Breast Cancer Detection Demonstration Project involving over 280,000 women showed that women exposed to estrogen for longer durations had increased risk for breast cancer [37–39]. Women who reached menarche before age 12 had increased risk of 1.3 compared with those with menarche after age 15, and women who reached menopause after the age of 55 had increased risk of 1.22 compared with those who reached menopause before 45. Also, women who underwent ovariectomy before age 40 showed a 45% reduction in breast cancer risk [39]. Another line of evidence is from chemoprevention studies that demonstrate how estrogen contributes to breast cancer carcinogenesis (Table 8.6). Randomized trials have been conducted to clarify the preventive effects of selective estrogen receptor modulators (SERMs) and aromatase inhibitors (Table 8.6). Randomized trials were conducted for comparison of tamoxifen and placebo groups in the National Surgical Adjuvant Breast and Bowel Project (NSABP P-1) [40], Royal Marsden [41], Italian Tamoxifen Prevention [42, 43], and IBIS-1 [44] trials. Others include exemestane and placebo groups in the MAP.3 trial [45]; raloxifene and placebo groups in the MORE [46], CORE [47], and RUTH [48] trials; lasofoxifene and placebo groups in the PEARL trial [49]; arzoxifene and placebo groups in the Generations trial [50]; anastrozole and placebo groups in the IBIS-II trial [51]; and raloxifene and tamoxifen groups in the STAR trial [52]. The hazard ratio (HR) was 0.84 and 0.84 for tamoxifen in the Royal Marsden and Italian Tamoxifen Prevention Study trials, respectively. The HR was 0.47 for exemestane in the MAP.3 trial and 0.38, 0.42, and 0.67 for raloxifene in the MORE, CORE, and RUTH trials, respectively. Also, the HR was 0.21 for lasofoxifene in the PEARL trial, 0.41 for arzoxifene in the Generations trial, and 0.47 for anastrozole in the IBIS-II trial. The results of these randomized trials indicate that SERMs and aromatase inhibitors had preventive effects.

Despite these supportive clinical data showing that carcinogenesis of breast cancer is related to estrogens (estrone, E1; estradiol, E2; estriol, E3), it is difficult to explain the mechanism of carcinogenesis in a simplified or straightforward manner. Epithelial cells expressing estrogen receptors (ER) receive signals from the estrogen-estrogen receptor (E-ER) axis. In the normal mammary gland, expression of

Table 8.6 Chemoprevention study

Trial	Number of patients	Hazard ratio (95% CI)		
		All breast cancer	Invasive breast cancer	DCIS
Tamoxifen and placebo				
NSABP P1, 2005 [40]	13,388	NR	0.57 (0.46–0.70)	0.63 (0.45–0.89)
Royal Marsden, 2007 [41]	2471	0.84 (0.64–1.10)	0.78 (0.58–1.04)	NR
ITPS, 1998 [42, 43]	5408	0.84 (0.60–1.17)	0.80 (0.56–1.15)	1.50 (0.53–4.20)
IBIS-I, 2011 [44]	1065	NR	NR	NR
Exemestane and placebo				
MAPs.3, 2011 [45]	4560	0.47 (0.27–0.79)	0.35 (0.18–0.70)	NR
Raloxifene and placebo				
MORE, 2001 [46]	7705	0.38 (0.24–0.58)	0.28 (0.17–0.46)	0.90 (0.30–2.69)
CORE, 2004 [47]	7705	0.42 (0.29–0.60)	0.34 (0.22–0.50)	1.12 (0.46–2.73)
RUTH, 2006 [48]	10,101	0.67 (0.47–0.96)	0.56 (0.38–0.83)	2.17 (0.75–6.24)
Lasofoxifene and placebo				
PEARL, 2010 [49]	5704	0.21 (0.08–0.55)	0.17 (0.05–0.57)	0.50 (0.09–2.73)
Arzoxifene and placebo				
Generations, 2012 [50]	9354	0.41 (0.25–0.68)	0.44 (0.26–0.76)	0.30 (0.08–1.09)
Anastrozole and placebo				
IBIS-II, 2014 [51]	3864	0.47 (0.32–0.68)	0.50 (0.32–0.76)	0.30 (0.12–0.74)
Raloxifene and tamoxifen				
STAR, 2010 [52]	19,471	NR	1.24 (1.05–1.47)	1.22 (0.95–1.59)

NSABP National Surgical Adjuvant Breast and Bowel Project; *ITPS* Italian Tamoxifen Prevention Study; *MORE* Multiple Outcomes for Raloxifene Examination; *CORE* Continuing Outcomes Relevant to Evista [raloxifene]; *RUTH* Raloxifene Use for The Heart; *STAR* Study for Tamoxifen and Raloxifene

ERα is not so high. ERα-positive cells in the normal mammary gland were detected in 4.0% [53], 7.0% [54], 17.3% [55], and 5–28% (around 10%) [56] of epithelial cells. Li et al. reported that ERα-positive cells were detected in epithelial cells at acini and in epithelial, myoepithelial, and stromal cells at the interlobular ducts [56]. The incidence of ERα-positive cases with various thresholds in each study was 0–57% [57–66] (Table 8.4). The ERα gene is usually unmethylated, or if methylated, it is expressed at low levels in the normal mammary gland [67–69] (Table 8.7); this lower expression of ERα gene is not considered to be due to hypermethylation. The expression of ERα in breast cancer is more monotonous, and the incidence of ERα-positive breast cancer was 31.5–61.5% [55, 58, 64]. In Japan, with the increased sensitivity of immunohistochemistry in the 1990s, and with the current aging population, the current incidence of ERα-positive breast cancer is approximately 70–75% [70–72].

A second ER, ERβ, was discovered in 1996 in rat prostate and ovary [73], and the human ERβ gene was reported to be located on 14q22–24. Homology to the ERα gene was 17.5%, 97.0%, 30.0%, 59.1%, and 17.9% at the A/B (NH_2-terminal), C (DNA binding), D (hinge), E (ligand binding), and F domains, respectively [74]. There are four splice variants ERβ2, ERβ5, ERβδ5, and ERβins that differ at the A/B and E domains compared with wild-type ERβ (ERβ1). ERβ-positive cells were detected in 85% of epithelial cells in the normal mammary gland [53], in epithelial cells and stromal cells at acini, and in epithelial cells, myoepithelial cells, and stromal cells at the interlobular ducts. The incidence of ERβ-positive cases is obviously higher than ERα-positive cases, with more than 90% [61, 66] occurring in the unmethylated form [75] (Table 8.7). The biological roles of ERβ differ from those of ERα, and suppressive effects for proliferation in cancer cells were reported [76, 77]. Heterodimerization of ERα/ERβ is also suspected to have suppressive effects that may depend on variants of ERβ [78].

Table 8.7 Expression of ERα and ERβ in the normal mammary gland and breast cancer

ERα			
Percentage of positive cells			
In the mammary gland	In DCIS	In breast cancer	Reference
4.0%	0.7%		[53]
7.0%			[54]
17.3%		31.5%	[55]
Proportion of ERα-positive cases			
In the mammary gland	In DCIS	In breast cancer	
6%	31%		[62]
31%		61.4%	[58]
0%		61.5%	[64]
Incidence of methylation			
Unmethylated			[67, 115]
8.3%			[68]
ERβ			
Percentage of positive cells			
In the mammary gland	In DCIS	In breast cancer	
85%	3.0%		[53]
Proportion of ERα-positive cases			
In the mammary gland	In DCIS	In breast cancer	
94.3%		85%	[116]
93%		31%	[61]
Incidence of methylation			
Unmethylated			[75]

ERα and ERβ homo- or heterodimers serve to regulate proliferation and differentiation of epithelial cells via the E-ER axis. In the normal mammary gland, Clarke et al. showed that ERα-positive cells expressed the progesterone receptor gene but not markers of proliferation including BrdU and Ki67, and dividing cells were ERα-negative cells. Cell proliferation is controlled by ERα-positive cells and ERα-negative cells via a paracrine mechanism [55]. Clarke et al. also showed that dividing cells in the tumor are ERα-positive. In breast cancer cells, the mitogenic effects of estrogens have been explained by two different mechanisms [79]: estrogen can induce genomic effects via estrogen-responsive elements located in the promoter region of c-fos [80] and/or c-myc [81] to affect mitogenic activity involving G1 phase progression and estrogen can also mediate indirect effects on cyclin D1 gene transcription [82]. Regulation of cyclin D1 gene transcription is strictly maintained in a hormone-dependent manner, and correspondingly the cAMP response element in the promoter region of the cyclin D1 gene requires interaction with the AF-1 and AF-2 domains of ERα. Other non-genomic actions of estrogen via MAPK/ERK and PI-3 K/Akt signaling pathways have been evaluated [79].

Another interesting issue to address is whether estrogens have a role as procarcinogens that induce genetic damage. Endogenous estrogens have been classified as epigenetic nongenotoxic carcinogens because the estrogens E2 and E1 and their catechol metabolites did not induce genetic mutation in the Ames bacterial reversion assay [83–85], in Syrian hamster embryo cells [86–90], or in V79 Chinese hamster cells [85, 91, 92]. Despite this failure to induce genetic mutation, there has been substantive evidence from in vitro and in vivo rodent experimental systems showing that *o*-quinones generated from the metabolic redox cycling of catechol estrogens induce DNA damage [93, 94]. Free radical-mediated DNA damage by estrogens and their metabolites was found to be single-strand breaks, 8-hydroxylation of guanine bases, bulky DNA adducts, E2-induced malondialdehyde-DNA adducts, and estrogen-DNA adducts. The genotoxic effects of endogenous estrogens continue to be a significant issue investigated in specific and sensitive experimental systems [93, 94].

As described earlier, epithelial cells in the normal mammary gland show low expression levels of ERα and high expression levels of ERβ in the presence of proliferating ERα-negative cells. Prolonged exposure to estrogens stimulates proliferation of epithelial cells, and this may allow accumulation of genetic alterations. At some point in the time course, ERα-positive, ERβ-positive, and AR-positive carcinoma cells may acquire the ability to proliferate autonomously. Clonal selection and expansion of these cells may occur, and hormone-dependent breast carcinoma with monotonous expression of ERα and a high positive rate for ERβ and AR may ensue.

In terms of risk factors, ER expression in atypical hyperplasia is another vital question. It has been shown that ERα expression in atypical hyperplasia is not a risk factor [95]. In contrast, ERβ expression has been shown to be a risk factor in the normal mammary gland and in atypical hyperplasia [96]. ERβ expression in the normal mammary gland is over 90%, and lower ERβ expression increased the risk by twofold ($p < 0.01$) in the normal mammary gland and by 2.5-fold ($p = 0.006$) in atypical hyperplasia; this was evaluated by scoring the proportion of ERβ-positive cells, staining intensity, and the sum of these two factors for a total immunohistochemistry score.

8.5 Gene Alterations Due to Numerical or Structural Chromosomal Changes and Methylation Detected in the Morphologically Normal Mammary Gland

A body of evidence has been accumulated demonstrating that the nonneoplastic mammary gland harbors a considerable number of genetic alterations, even in the absence of morphological abnormalities. Danforth [97] reviewed the literature on molecular changes in normal breast tissue. The review categorized normal breast tissue into normal-risk and high-risk breast tissue. The former category included breast tissue obtained from women with no personal history of breast cancer or who had undergone reduction mammoplasty and from biopsies of benign or normal breast tissue. The latter category comprised normal breast tissue adjacent to atypical hyperplasia or malignant lesions, normal breast tissue in the contralateral breast of women with breast cancer, and normal breast tissue from women likely to develop breast cancer in the future. In this review, structural chromosomal changes were detected even in the normal breast tissue at normal risk, for example, loss of heterozygosity of 1q, 1p, 3p, 9p, 9q, 11p, 11q, 13q, 16q, 17p, and 17q. The normal breast tissue at high risk harbored increased number of numerical and structural chromosomal changes. Thus, mammary epithelial cells accumulate genetic alterations even in the early phase that cannot be detected as morphological changes.

Conclusion

Germline mutations of *BRCA1* and family history have been found to be high-risk factors, and atypical hyperplasia (ADH, ALH) was a significant risk factor with relative risk ranging from 3.93 to 5.0. The clinical and biological significance of estrogen exposure and expression of ER was reviewed and discussed. Finally, numerical and structural chromosomal alterations as well as epigenetic changes in the morphologically normal mammary gland were examined. Molecular investigation about the process from the normal-looking mammary gland harboring genetic alteration to breast carcinoma may reveal risk factors in addition to those that had been detected by epidemiological studies.

References

1. Hall JM, Lee MK, Newman B, Morrow JE, Anderson LA, Huey B, King MC. Linkage of early-onset familial breast cancer to chromosome 17q21. Science. 1990;250(4988):1684–9.
2. Narod SA, Feunteun J, Lynch HT, Watson P, Conway T, Lynch J, Lenoir GM. Familial breast-ovarian cancer locus on chromosome 17q12-q23. Lancet. 1991;338(8759):82–3.
3. Easton DF, Bishop DT, Ford D, Crockford GP. Genetic linkage analysis in familial breast and ovarian cancer: results from 214 families. The Breast Cancer Linkage Consortium. Am J Hum Genet. 1993;52(4):678–701.
4. Miki Y, Swensen J, Shattuck-Eidens D, Futreal PA, Harshman K, Tavtigian S, Liu Q, Cochran C, Bennett LM, Ding W, et al. A strong candidate for the breast and ovarian cancer susceptibility gene BRCA1. Science. 1994;266(5182):66–71.
5. Easton DF, Ford D, Bishop DT. Breast and ovarian cancer incidence in BRCA1-mutation carriers. Breast Cancer Linkage Consortium. Am J Hum Genet. 1995;56(1):265–71.
6. Antoniou A, Pharoah PD, Narod S, Risch HA, Eyfjord JE, Hopper JL, Loman N, Olsson H, Johannsson O, Borg A, Pasini B, Radice P, Manoukian S, Eccles DM, Tang N, Olah E, Anton-Culver H, Warner E, Lubinski J, Gronwald J, Gorski B, Tulinius H, Thorlacius S, Eerola H, Nevanlinna H, Syrjakoski K, Kallioniemi OP, Thompson D, Evans C, Peto J, Lalloo F, Evans DG, Easton DF. Average risks of breast and ovarian cancer associated with BRCA1 or BRCA2 mutations detected in case Series unselected for family history: a combined analysis of 22 studies. Am J Hum Genet. 2003;72(5):1117–30. https://doi.org/10.1086/375033.
7. Chen S, Parmigiani G. Meta-analysis of BRCA1 and BRCA2 penetrance. J Clin Oncol. 2007;25(11):1329–33. https://doi.org/10.1200/JCO.2006.09.1066.
8. Gail MH, Brinton LA, Byar DP, Corle DK, Green SB, Schairer C, Mulvihill JJ. Projecting individualized probabilities of developing breast cancer for white females who are being examined annually. J Natl Cancer Inst. 1989;81(24):1879–86.
9. Colditz GA, Rosner B. Cumulative risk of breast cancer to age 70 years according to risk factor status: data from the Nurses' Health Study. Am J Epidemiol. 2000;152(10):950–64.

10. Parmigiani G, Berry D, Aguilar O. Determining carrier probabilities for breast cancer-susceptibility genes BRCA1 and BRCA2. Am J Hum Genet. 1998;62(1):145–58.
11. Tyrer J, Duffy SW, Cuzick J. A breast cancer prediction model incorporating familial and personal risk factors. Stat Med. 2004;23(7):1111–30. https://doi.org/10.1002/sim.1668.
12. Antoniou AC, Pharoah PD, McMullan G, Day NE, Stratton MR, Peto J, Ponder BJ, Easton DF. A comprehensive model for familial breast cancer incorporating BRCA1, BRCA2 and other genes. Br J Cancer. 2002;86(1):76–83. https://doi.org/10.1038/sj.bjc.6600008.
13. Antoniou AC, Pharoah PP, Smith P, Easton DF. The BOADICEA model of genetic susceptibility to breast and ovarian cancer. Br J Cancer. 2004;91(8):1580–90. https://doi.org/10.1038/sj.bjc.6602175.
14. Antoniou AC, Cunningham AP, Peto J, Evans DG, Lalloo F, Narod SA, Risch HA, Eyfjord JE, Hopper JL, Southey MC, Olsson H, Johannsson O, Borg A, Pasini B, Radice P, Manoukian S, Eccles DM, Tang N, Olah E, Anton-Culver H, Warner E, Lubinski J, Gronwald J, Gorski B, Tryggvadottir L, Syrjakoski K, Kallioniemi OP, Eerola H, Nevanlinna H, Pharoah PD, Easton DF. The BOADICEA model of genetic susceptibility to breast and ovarian cancers: updates and extensions. Br J Cancer. 2008;98(8):1457–66. https://doi.org/10.1038/sj.bjc.6604305.
15. Claus EB, Risch N, Thompson WD. Autosomal dominant inheritance of early-onset breast cancer. Implications for risk prediction. Cancer. 1994;73(3):643–51.
16. Hoda SA. "Ductal hyperplasia: usual and atypical" in Hoda SA, Brogi E, Koerner FC, Rosen PP eds. Rosen's breast pathology 4th ed., Woters Kluwer, Philadelphia;2014. p. 271–307.
17. Page DL, Dupont WD, Rogers LW, Rados MS. Atypical hyperplastic lesions of the female breast. A long-term follow-up study. Cancer. 1985;55(11):2698–708.
18. Tavassoli FA, Norris HJ. A comparison of the results of long-term follow-up for atypical intraductal hyperplasia and intraductal hyperplasia of the breast. Cancer. 1990;65(3):518–29.
19. Hartmann LC, Sellers TA, Frost MH, Lingle WL, Degnim AC, Ghosh K, Vierkant RA, Maloney SD, Pankratz VS, Hillman DW, Suman VJ, Johnson J, Blake C, Tlsty T, Vachon CM, Melton LJ III, Visscher DW. Benign breast disease and the risk of breast cancer. N Engl J Med. 2005;353(3):229–37. https://doi.org/10.1056/NEJMoa044383.
20. London SJ, Connolly JL, Schnitt SJ, Colditz GA. A prospective study of benign breast disease and the risk of breast cancer. JAMA. 1992;267(7):941–4.
21. Worsham MJ, Raju U, Lu M, Kapke A, Cheng J, Wolman SR. Multiplicity of benign breast lesions is a risk factor for progression to breast cancer. Clin Cancer Res. 2007;13(18 Pt 1):5474–9. https://doi.org/10.1158/1078-0432.CCR-07-0928.
22. Moriya T, Kasami M, Akiyama F, Ichihara S, Kurosumi M, Tsuda H, Umemura S, Akashi-Tanaka S, Imamura H, Iwase H, Shin E, Harada Y, Mitsuyama S, Ohuchi N. A proposal for the histopathological diagnosis of ductal carcinoma in situ of the breast. Breast Cancer. 2000;7(4):321–5.
23. Chuba PJ, Hamre MR, Yap J, Severson RK, Lucas D, Shamsa F, Aref A. Bilateral risk for subsequent breast cancer after lobular carcinoma-in-situ: analysis of surveillance, epidemiology, and end results data. J Clin Oncol. 2005;23(24):5534–41. https://doi.org/10.1200/JCO.2005.04.038.
24. Degnim AC, Visscher DW, Berman HK, Frost MH, Sellers TA, Vierkant RA, Maloney SD, Pankratz VS, de Groen PC, Lingle WL, Ghosh K, Penheiter L, Tlsty T, Melton LJ III, Reynolds CA, Hartmann LC. Stratification of breast cancer risk in women with atypia: a Mayo cohort study. J Clin Oncol. 2007;25(19):2671–7. https://doi.org/10.1200/JCO.2006.09.0217.
25. Degnim AC, Dupont WD, Radisky DC, Vierkant RA, Frank RD, Frost MH, Winham SJ, Sanders ME, Smith JR, Page DL, Hoskin TL, Vachon CM, Ghosh K, Hieken TJ, Denison LA, Carter JM, Hartmann LC, Visscher DW. Extent of atypical hyperplasia stratifies breast cancer risk in 2 independent cohorts of women. Cancer. 2016;122(19):2971–8. https://doi.org/10.1002/cncr.30153.
26. Collins LC, Aroner SA, Connolly JL, Colditz GA, Schnitt SJ, Tamimi RM. Breast cancer risk by extent and type of atypical hyperplasia: an update from the Nurses' Health Studies. Cancer. 2016;122(4):515–20. https://doi.org/10.1002/cncr.29775.
27. Degnim AC, Visscher DW, Radisky DC, Frost MH, Vierkant RA, Frank RD, Winham SJ, Vachon CM, Dupont WD, Hartmann LC. Breast cancer risk by the extent and type of atypical hyperplasia. Cancer. 2016;122(19):3087–8. https://doi.org/10.1002/cncr.30151.
28. Collins LC, Schnitt SJ, Tamimi RM. Reply to breast cancer risk by the extent and type of atypical hyperplasia. Cancer. 2016;122(19):3088–9. https://doi.org/10.1002/cncr.30149.
29. Said SM, Visscher DW, Nassar A, Frank RD, Vierkant RA, Frost MH, Ghosh K, Radisky DC, Hartmann LC, Degnim AC. Flat epithelial atypia and risk of breast cancer: a Mayo cohort study. Cancer. 2015;121(10):1548–55. https://doi.org/10.1002/cncr.29243.
30. Visscher DW, Nassar A, Degnim AC, Frost MH, Vierkant RA, Frank RD, Tarabishy Y, Radisky DC, Hartmann LC. Sclerosing adenosis and risk of breast cancer. Breast Cancer Res Treat. 2014;144(1):205–12. https://doi.org/10.1007/s10549-014-2862-5.
31. Hamperl H. Radial scars (scarring) and obliterating mastopathy (author's transl). Virchows Arch A Pathol Anat Histol. 1975;369(1):55–68.
32. Berg JC, Visscher DW, Vierkant RA, Pankratz VS, Maloney SD, Lewis JT, Frost MH, Ghosh K, Degnim AC, Brandt KR, Vachon CM, Reynolds CA, Hartmann LC. Breast cancer risk in women with radial scars in benign breast biopsies. Breast Cancer Res Treat. 2008;108(2):167–74. https://doi.org/10.1007/s10549-007-9605-9.
33. Rosen PP. Mucocele-like tumors of the breast. Am J Surg Pathol. 1986;10(7):464–9.
34. Hamele-Bena D, Cranor ML, Rosen PP. Mammary mucocele-like lesions. Benign and malignant. Am J Surg Pathol. 1996;20(9):1081–5.
35. Meares AL, Frank RD, Degnim AC, Vierkant RA, Frost MH, Hartmann LC, Winham SJ, Visscher DW. Mucocele-like lesions of the breast: a clinical outcome and histologic analysis of 102 cases. Hum Pathol. 2016;49:33–8. https://doi.org/10.1016/j.humpath.2015.10.004.
36. Trichopoulos D, MacMahon B, Cole P. Menopause and breast cancer risk. J Natl Cancer Inst. 1972;48(3):605–13.
37. Brinton LA, Hoover R, Fraumeni JF Jr. Reproductive factors in the aetiology of breast cancer. Br J Cancer. 1983;47(6):757–62.
38. Brinton LA, Hoover R, Fraumeni JF Jr. Epidemiology of minimal breast cancer. JAMA. 1983;249(4):483–7.
39. Brinton LA, Schairer C, Hoover RN, Fraumeni JF Jr. Menstrual factors and risk of breast cancer. Cancer Investig. 1988;6(3):245–54.
40. Fisher B, Costantino JP, Wickerham DL, Cecchini RS, Cronin WM, Robidoux A, Bevers TB, Kavanah MT, Atkins JN, Margolese RG, Runowicz CD, James JM, Ford LG, Wolmark N. Tamoxifen for the prevention of breast cancer: current status of the National Surgical Adjuvant Breast and Bowel Project P-1 study. J Natl Cancer Inst. 2005;97(22):1652–62. https://doi.org/10.1093/jnci/dji372.
41. Powles TJ, Ashley S, Tidy A, Smith IE, Dowsett M. Twenty-year follow-up of the Royal Marsden randomized, double-blinded tamoxifen breast cancer prevention trial. J Natl Cancer Inst. 2007;99(4):283–90. https://doi.org/10.1093/jnci/djk050.
42. Veronesi U, Maisonneuve P, Costa A, Sacchini V, Maltoni C, Robertson C, Rotmensz N, Boyle P. Prevention of breast cancer with tamoxifen: preliminary findings from the Italian randomised trial among hysterectomised women. Italian Tamoxifen Prevention Study. Lancet. 1998;352(9122):93–7.

43. Cuzick J, Sestak I, Bonanni B, Costantino JP, Cummings S, DeCensi A, Dowsett M, Forbes JF, Ford L, LaCroix AZ, Mershon J, Mitlak BH, Powles T, Veronesi U, Vogel V, Wickerham DL, Group SCoBCO. Selective oestrogen receptor modulators in prevention of breast cancer: an updated meta-analysis of individual participant data. Lancet. 2013;381(9880):1827–34. https://doi.org/10.1016/S0140-6736(13)60140-3.
44. Cuzick J, Warwick J, Pinney E, Duffy SW, Cawthorn S, Howell A, Forbes JF, Warren RM. Tamoxifen-induced reduction in mammographic density and breast cancer risk reduction: a nested case-control study. J Natl Cancer Inst. 2011;103(9):744–52. https://doi.org/10.1093/jnci/djr079.
45. Goss PE, Ingle JN, Ales-Martinez JE, Cheung AM, Chlebowski RT, Wactawski-Wende J, McTiernan A, Robbins J, Johnson KC, Martin LW, Winquist E, Sarto GE, Garber JE, Fabian CJ, Pujol P, Maunsell E, Farmer P, Gelmon KA, Tu D, Richardson H, Investigators NCMS. Exemestane for breast-cancer prevention in postmenopausal women. N Engl J Med. 2011;364(25):2381–91. https://doi.org/10.1056/NEJMoa1103507.
46. Cauley JA, Norton L, Lippman ME, Eckert S, Krueger KA, Purdie DW, Farrerons J, Karasik A, Mellstrom D, Ng KW, Stepan JJ, Powles TJ, Morrow M, Costa A, Silfen SL, Walls EL, Schmitt H, Muchmore DB, Jordan VC, Ste-Marie LG. Continued breast cancer risk reduction in postmenopausal women treated with raloxifene: 4-year results from the MORE trial. Multiple outcomes of raloxifene evaluation. Breast Cancer Res Treat. 2001;65(2):125–34.
47. Martino S, Cauley JA, Barrett-Connor E, Powles TJ, Mershon J, Disch D, Secrest RJ, Cummings SR, Investigators C. Continuing outcomes relevant to Evista: breast cancer incidence in postmenopausal osteoporotic women in a randomized trial of raloxifene. J Natl Cancer Inst. 2004;96(23):1751–61. https://doi.org/10.1093/jnci/djh319.
48. Barrett-Connor E, Mosca L, Collins P, Geiger MJ, Grady D, Kornitzer M, McNabb MA, Wenger NK, Raloxifene Use for The Heart Trial I. Effects of raloxifene on cardiovascular events and breast cancer in postmenopausal women. N Engl J Med. 2006;355(2):125–37. https://doi.org/10.1056/NEJMoa062462.
49. LaCroix AZ, Powles T, Osborne CK, Wolter K, Thompson JR, Thompson DD, Allred DC, Armstrong R, Cummings SR, Eastell R, Ensrud KE, Goss P, Lee A, Neven P, Reid DM, Curto M, Vukicevic S, Investigators P. Breast cancer incidence in the randomized PEARL trial of lasofoxifene in postmenopausal osteoporotic women. J Natl Cancer Inst. 2010;102(22):1706–15. https://doi.org/10.1093/jnci/djq415.
50. Powles TJ, Diem SJ, Fabian CJ, Neven P, Wickerham DL, Cox DA, Muram D, Agnusdei D, Dowsett SA, Amewou-Atisso M, Cummings SR. Breast cancer incidence in postmenopausal women with osteoporosis or low bone mass using arzoxifene. Breast Cancer Res Treat. 2012;134(1):299–306. https://doi.org/10.1007/s10549-012-2041-5.
51. Cuzick J, Sestak I, Forbes JF, Dowsett M, Knox J, Cawthorn S, Saunders C, Roche N, Mansel RE, von Minckwitz G, Bonanni B, Palva T, Howell A, investigators I-I. Anastrozole for prevention of breast cancer in high-risk postmenopausal women (IBIS-II): an international, double-blind, randomised placebo-controlled trial. Lancet. 2014;383(9922):1041–8. https://doi.org/10.1016/S0140-6736(13)62292-8.
52. Vogel VG, Costantino JP, Wickerham DL, Cronin WM, Cecchini RS, Atkins JN, Bevers TB, Fehrenbacher L, Pajon ER, Wade JL 3rd, Robidoux A, Margolese RG, James J, Runowicz CD, Ganz PA, Reis SE, McCaskill-Stevens W, Ford LG, Jordan VC, Wolmark N, National Surgical Adjuvant B, Bowel P. Update of the National Surgical Adjuvant Breast and Bowel Project Study of Tamoxifen and Raloxifene (STAR) P-2 Trial: preventing breast cancer. Cancer Prev Res (Phila). 2010;3(6):696–706. https://doi.org/10.1158/1940-6207.CAPR-10-0076.
53. Roger P, Sahla ME, Makela S, Gustafsson JA, Baldet P, Rochefort H. Decreased expression of estrogen receptor beta protein in proliferative preinvasive mammary tumors. Cancer Res. 2001;61(6):2537–41.
54. Petersen OW, Hoyer PE, van Deurs B. Frequency and distribution of estrogen receptor-positive cells in normal, nonlactating human breast tissue. Cancer Res. 1987;47(21):5748–51.
55. Clarke RB, Howell A, Potten CS, Anderson E. Dissociation between steroid receptor expression and cell proliferation in the human breast. Cancer Res. 1997;57(22):4987–91.
56. Li S, Han B, Liu G, Li S, Ouellet J, Labrie F, Pelletier G. Immunocytochemical localization of sex steroid hormone receptors in normal human mammary gland. J Histochem Cytochem. 2010;58(6):509–15. https://doi.org/10.1369/jhc.2009.954644.
57. Battersby S, Robertson BJ, Anderson TJ, King RJ, McPherson K. Influence of menstrual cycle, parity and oral contraceptive use on steroid hormone receptors in normal breast. Br J Cancer. 1992;65(4):601–7.
58. Markopoulos C, Berger U, Wilson P, Gazet JC, Coombes RC. Oestrogen receptor content of normal breast cells and breast carcinomas throughout the menstrual cycle. Br Med J (Clin Res Ed). 1988;296(6633):1349–51.
59. Shoker BS, Jarvis C, Clarke RB, Anderson E, Hewlett J, Davies MP, Sibson DR, Sloane JP. Estrogen receptor-positive proliferating cells in the normal and precancerous breast. Am J Pathol. 1999;155(6):1811–5. https://doi.org/10.1016/S0002-9440(10)65498-3.
60. Shoker BS, Jarvis C, Clarke RB, Anderson E, Munro C, Davies MP, Sibson DR, Sloane JP. Abnormal regulation of the oestrogen receptor in benign breast lesions. J Clin Pathol. 2000;53(10):778–83.
61. Abdel-Fatah TM, Powe DG, Hodi Z, Reis-Filho JS, Lee AH, Ellis IO. Morphologic and molecular evolutionary pathways of low nuclear grade invasive breast cancers and their putative precursor lesions: further evidence to support the concept of low nuclear grade breast neoplasia family. Am J Surg Pathol. 2008;32(4):513–23. https://doi.org/10.1097/PAS.0b013e318161d1a5.
62. Jacquemier JD, Hassoun J, Torrente M, Martin PM. Distribution of estrogen and progesterone receptors in healthy tissue adjacent to breast lesions at various stages—immunohistochemical study of 107 cases. Breast Cancer Res Treat. 1990;15(2):109–17.
63. Ricketts D, Turnbull L, Ryall G, Bakhshi R, Rawson NS, Gazet JC, Nolan C, Coombes RC. Estrogen and progesterone receptors in the normal female breast. Cancer Res. 1991;51(7):1817–22.
64. Netto GJ, Cheek JH, Zachariah NY, Romer JC, Lee CF, Schoenfeld R, Chakmakjian ZH. Steroid receptors in benign mastectomy tissue. Am J Clin Pathol. 1990;94(1):14–7.
65. Fabian CJ, Zalles C, Kamel S, Kimler BF, McKittrick R, Tranin AS, Zeiger S, Moore WP, Hassanein RS, Simon C, et al. Prevalence of aneuploidy, overexpressed ER, and overexpressed EGFR in random breast aspirates of women at high and low risk for breast cancer. Breast Cancer Res Treat. 1994;30(3):263–74.
66. Khan SA, Rogers MA, Obando JA, Tamsen A. Estrogen receptor expression of benign breast epithelium and its association with breast cancer. Cancer Res. 1994;54(4):993–7.
67. Wei M, Xu J, Dignam J, Nanda R, Sveen L, Fackenthal J, Grushko TA, Olopade OI. Estrogen receptor alpha, BRCA1, and FANCF promoter methylation occur in distinct subsets of sporadic breast cancers. Breast Cancer Res Treat. 2008;111(1):113–20. https://doi.org/10.1007/s10549-007-9766-6.
68. Jeronimo C, Monteiro P, Henrique R, Dinis-Ribeiro M, Costa I, Costa VL, Filipe L, Carvalho AL, Hoque MO, Pais I, Leal C, Teixeira MR, Sidransky D. Quantitative hypermethylation of a small panel of genes augments the diagnostic accuracy in fine-needle aspirate washings of breast lesions. Breast Cancer Res Treat. 2008;109(1):27–34. https://doi.org/10.1007/s10549-007-9620-x.

69. Lapidus RG, Nass SJ, Butash KA, Parl FF, Weitzman SA, Graff JG, Herman JG, Davidson NE. Mapping of ER gene CpG island methylation-specific polymerase chain reaction. Cancer Res. 1998;58(12):2515–9.
70. Iwamoto T, Fukui N, Kinoshita T, Anan K, Niikura N, Kawai M, Hayashi N, Tsugawa K, Aogi K, Ishida T, Masuoka H, Masuda S, Iijima K, Nakamura S, Tokuda Y. Comprehensive prognostic report of the Japanese Breast Cancer Society registry in 2006. Breast Cancer. 2015;23:62. https://doi.org/10.1007/s12282-015-0646-3.
71. Anan K, Fukui N, Kinoshita T, Iwamoto T, Niikura N, Kawai M, Hayashi N, Tsugawa K, Aogi K, Ishida T, Masuoka H, Masuda S, Iijima K, Nakamura S, Tokuda Y. Comprehensive prognostic report of the Japanese Breast Cancer Society Registry in 2005. Breast Cancer. 2015;23:50. https://doi.org/10.1007/s12282-015-0645-4.
72. Kinoshita T, Fukui N, Anan K, Iwamoto T, Niikura N, Kawai M, Hayashi N, Tsugawa K, Aogi K, Ishida T, Masuoka H, Masuda S, Iijima K, Nakamura S, Tokuda Y. Comprehensive prognostic report of the Japanese Breast Cancer Society Registry in 2004. Breast Cancer. 2016;23(1):39–49. https://doi.org/10.1007/s12282-015-0644-5.
73. Kuiper GG, Enmark E, Pelto-Huikko M, Nilsson S, Gustafsson JA. Cloning of a novel receptor expressed in rat prostate and ovary. Proc Natl Acad Sci U S A. 1996;93(12):5925–30.
74. Enmark E. Human estrogen receptor-gene structure, chromosomal localization, and expression pattern. J Clin Endocrinol Metab. 1997;82(12):4258–65. https://doi.org/10.1210/jc.82.12.4258.
75. Rody A, Holtrich U, Solbach C, Kourtis K, von Minckwitz G, Engels K, Kissler S, Gatje R, Karn T, Kaufmann M. Methylation of estrogen receptor beta promoter correlates with loss of ER-beta expression in mammary carcinoma and is an early indication marker in premalignant lesions. Endocr Relat Cancer. 2005;12(4):903–16. https://doi.org/10.1677/erc.1.01088.
76. Lazennec G, Bresson D, Lucas A, Chauveau C, Vignon F. ER beta inhibits proliferation and invasion of breast cancer cells. Endocrinology. 2001;142(9):4120–30. https://doi.org/10.1210/endo.142.9.8395.
77. Paruthiyil S, Parmar H, Kerekatte V, Cunha GR, Firestone GL, Leitman DC. Estrogen receptor beta inhibits human breast cancer cell proliferation and tumor formation by causing a G2 cell cycle arrest. Cancer Res. 2004;64(1):423–8.
78. Higa GM, Fell RG. Sex hormone receptor repertoire in breast cancer. Int J Breast Cancer. 2013;2013:284036. https://doi.org/10.1155/2013/284036.
79. Gaben AM, Saucier C, Bedin M, Redeuilh G, Mester J. Mitogenic activity of estrogens in human breast cancer cells does not rely on direct induction of mitogen-activated protein kinase/extracellularly regulated kinase or phosphatidylinositol 3-kinase. Mol Endocrinol. 2004;18(11):2700–13. https://doi.org/10.1210/me.2003-0133.
80. Weisz A, Rosales R. Identification of an estrogen response element upstream of the human c-fos gene that binds the estrogen receptor and the AP-1 transcription factor. Nucleic Acids Res. 1990;18(17):5097–106.
81. Dubik D, Shiu RP. Mechanism of estrogen activation of c-myc oncogene expression. Oncogene. 1992;7(8):1587–94.
82. Sabbah M, Courilleau D, Mester J, Redeuilh G. Estrogen induction of the cyclin D1 promoter: involvement of a cAMP response-like element. Proc Natl Acad Sci U S A. 1999;96(20):11217–22.
83. Lang R, Redmann U. Non-mutagenicity of some sex hormones in the Ames salmonella/microsome mutagenicity test. Mutat Res. 1979;67(4):361–5.
84. Liehr JG, Fang WF, Sirbasku DA, Ari-Ulubelen A. Carcinogenicity of catechol estrogens in Syrian hamsters. J Steroid Biochem. 1986;24(1):353–6.
85. Lang R, Reimann R. Studies for a genotoxic potential of some endogenous and exogenous sex steroids. I. Communication: examination for the induction of gene mutations using the Ames Salmonella/microsome test and the HGPRT test in V79 cells. Environ Mol Mutagen. 1993;21(3):272–304.
86. Barrett JC, Wong A, McLachlan JA. Diethylstilbestrol induces neoplastic transformation without measurable gene mutation at two loci. Science. 1981;212(4501):1402–4.
87. Tsutsui T, Maizumi H, McLachlan JA, Barrett JC. Aneuploidy induction and cell transformation by diethylstilbestrol: a possible chromosomal mechanism in carcinogenesis. Cancer Res. 1983;43(8):3814–21.
88. Tsutsui T, Suzuki N, Fukuda S, Sato M, Maizumi H, McLachlan JA, Barrett JC. 17beta-Estradiol-induced cell transformation and aneuploidy of Syrian hamster embryo cells in culture. Carcinogenesis. 1987;8(11):1715–9.
89. Barrett JC, Tsutsui T. Mechanisms of estrogen-associated carcinogenesis. Prog Clin Biol Res. 1996;394:105–11.
90. Tsutsui T, Barrett JC. Neoplastic transformation of cultured mammalian cells by estrogens and estrogenlike chemicals. Environ Health Perspect. 1997;105(Suppl 3):619–24.
91. Drevon C, Piccoli C, Montesano R. Mutagenicity assays of estrogenic hormones in mammalian cells. Mutat Res. 1981;89(1):83–90.
92. Rajah TT, Pento JT. The mutagenic potential of antiestrogens at the HPRT locus in V79 cells. Res Commun Mol Pathol Pharmacol. 1995;89(1):85–92.
93. Liehr JG. Is estradiol a genotoxic mutagenic carcinogen? Endocr Rev. 2000;21(1):40–54. https://doi.org/10.1210/edrv.21.1.0386.
94. Roy D, Liehr JG. Estrogen, DNA damage and mutations. Mutat Res. 1999;424(1–2):107–15.
95. Barr FE, Degnim AC, Hartmann LC, Radisky DC, Boughey JC, Anderson SS, Vierkant RA, Frost MH, Visscher DW, Reynolds C. Estrogen receptor expression in atypical hyperplasia: lack of association with breast cancer. Cancer Prev Res (Phila). 2011; 4(3):435–44. https://doi.org/10.1158/1940-6207.CAPR-10-0242.
96. Hieken TJ, Carter JM, Hawse JR, Hoskin TL, Bois M, Frost M, Hartmann LC, Radisky DC, Visscher DW, Degnim AC. ERbeta expression and breast cancer risk prediction for women with atypias. Cancer Prev Res (Phila). 2015;8(11):1084–92. https://doi.org/10.1158/1940-6207.CAPR-15-0198.
97. Danforth DN Jr. Genomic changes in normal breast tissue in women at normal risk or at high risk for breast cancer. Breast Cancer (Auckl). 2016;10:109–46. https://doi.org/10.4137/BCBCR.S39384.
98. Pharoah PD, Day NE, Duffy S, Easton DF, Ponder BA. Family history and the risk of breast cancer: a systematic review and meta-analysis. Int J Cancer. 1997;71(5):800–9.
99. Ellison RC, Zhang Y, McLennan CE, Rothman KJ. Exploring the relation of alcohol consumption to risk of breast cancer. Am J Epidemiol. 2001;154(8):740–7.
100. Tretli S. Height and weight in relation to breast cancer morbidity and mortality. A prospective study of 570,000 women in Norway. Int J Cancer. 1989;44(1):23–30.
101. Nelson HD, Humphrey LL, Nygren P, Teutsch SM, Allan JD. Postmenopausal hormone replacement therapy: scientific review. JAMA. 2002;288(7):872–81.
102. Ries AL. SEER cancer statistics review, 1973–1997. Bethesda, MD: National Cancer Institute. NIH; 2000.
103. White E. Projected changes in breast cancer incidence due to the trend toward delayed childbearing. Am J Public Health. 1987;77(4):495–7.
104. Hankey BF, Curtis RE, Naughton MD, Boice JD Jr, Flannery JT. A retrospective cohort analysis of second breast cancer risk for primary breast cancer patients with an assessment of the effect of radiation therapy. J Natl Cancer Inst. 1983;70(5):797–804.
105. Rosen PP, Groshen S, Kinne DW, Hellman S. Contralateral breast carcinoma: an assessment of risk and prognosis in stage I (T1N0M0) and stage II (T1N1M0) patients with 20-year follow-up. Surgery. 1989;106(5):904–10.

106. Styblo TM, Wood WC. The management of ductal and lobular breast cancer. Surg Oncol. 1999;8(2):67–75.
107. Page DL, Dupont WD, Rogers LW, Landenberger M. Intraductal carcinoma of the breast: follow-up after biopsy only. Cancer. 1982;49(4):751–8.
108. Dupont WD, Parl FF, Hartmann WH, Brinton LA, Winfield AC, Worrell JA, Schuyler PA, Plummer WD. Breast cancer risk associated with proliferative breast disease and atypical hyperplasia. Cancer. 1993;71(4):1258–65.
109. Boice JD Jr, Preston D, Davis FG, Monson RR. Frequent chest X-ray fluoroscopy and breast cancer incidence among tuberculosis patients in Massachusetts. Radiat Res. 1991;125(2):214–22.
110. Clemons M, Loijens L, Goss P. Breast cancer risk following irradiation for Hodgkin's disease. Cancer Treat Rev. 2000;26(4):291–302. https://doi.org/10.1053/ctrv.2000.0174.
111. Hartmann LC, Degnim AC, Santen RJ, Dupont WD, Ghosh K. Atypical hyperplasia of the breast—risk assessment and management options. N Engl J Med. 2015;372(1):78–89. https://doi.org/10.1056/NEJMsr1407164.
112. Worsham MJ, Abrams J, Raju U, Kapke A, Lu M, Cheng J, Mott D, Wolman SR. Breast cancer incidence in a cohort of women with benign breast disease from a multiethnic, primary health care population. Breast J. 2007;13(2):115–21. https://doi.org/10.1111/j.1524-4741.2007.00388.x.
113. Hartmann LC, Radisky DC, Frost MH, Santen RJ, Vierkant RA, Benetti LL, Tarabishy Y, Ghosh K, Visscher DW, Degnim AC. Understanding the premalignant potential of atypical hyperplasia through its natural history: a longitudinal cohort study. Cancer Prev Res (Phila). 2014;7(2):211–7. https://doi.org/10.1158/1940-6207.CAPR-13-0222.
114. Collins LC, Baer HJ, Tamimi RM, Connolly JL, Colditz GA, Schnitt SJ. The influence of family history on breast cancer risk in women with biopsy-confirmed benign breast disease: results from the Nurses' Health Study. Cancer. 2006;107(6):1240–7. https://doi.org/10.1002/cncr.22136.
115. Lapidus RG, Nass SJ, Davidson NE. The loss of estrogen and progesterone receptor gene expression in human breast cancer. J Mammary Gland Biol Neoplasia. 1998;3(1):85–94.
116. Shaaban AM, O'Neill PA, Davies MP, Sibson R, West CR, Smith PH, Foster CS. Declining estrogen receptor-beta expression defines malignant progression of human breast neoplasia. Am J Surg Pathol. 2003;27(12):1502–12.

MIX
Papier aus verantwortungsvollen Quellen
Paper from responsible sources
FSC® C105338

If you have any concerns about our products,
you can contact us on
ProductSafety@springernature.com

In case Publisher is established outside the EU,
the EU authorized representative is:
Springer Nature Customer Service Center GmbH
Europaplatz 3, 69115 Heidelberg, Germany

Printed by Libri Plureos GmbH
in Hamburg, Germany